Promoting Effective Contraceptive Use

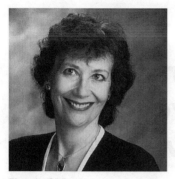

Photo by Gil Brady.

Dona J. Lethbridge, PhD, RN, received a diploma in nursing from the Royal Columbian Hospital School of Nursing, a BScN from the University of British Columbia, and a MA and PhD in nursing from New York University. She completed a post-doctoral fellowship at the University of Washington in women's health research, focusing on qualitative and feminist research methodologies, and the implications of class, ethnicity, and gender on research. She is currently an associate professor and research facilitator at the University of Alabama in Huntsville College of Nursing. Her research and clinical interests have focused on maternal–child nursing and women's health, with emphasis on contraceptive use. Her current work concerns these issues and the status of health in general, in very low-income, rural women. She has written extensively and spoken nationally and internationally on all of these topics.

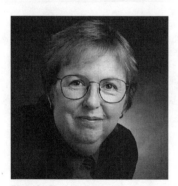

Photo by Paul K. Jacques.

Kathleen M. Hanna, PhD, RN, received a diploma from West Nebraska General Hospital School of Nursing, a BS in Nursing from Loretto Heights College, an MSN in Nursing from the University of Nebraska Medical Center, and a PhD in Nursing from the University of Pittsburgh. The focus of her graduate studies was parent–child nursing. Clinical experience has included nursing of children and adolescents in acute care and ambulatory settings, including family-planning clinics. Her research interests are in the area of adolescents' health beliefs and behaviors, with a specific interest in contraceptive behaviors. Currently, Dr. Hanna is studying adolescents' beliefs about and use of hormonal contraceptives and condoms. Her writings and presentations have been in both the broad area of adolescents' health and the specific area of adolescents' use of contraception. She is currently Assistant Professor in the School of Nursing at the University of Wyoming.

Promoting Effective Contraceptive Use

Dona J. Lethbridge, PhD, RN
Kathleen M. Hanna, PhD, RN

Springer Publishing Company

Springer Publishing Company, Inc.
536 Broadway
New York, NY 10012-3955

Cover design by Margaret Dunin
Production Editor: Pamela Lankas

97 98 99 00 01 / 5 4 3 2 1

Library of Congress Cataloging-in-Publication-Data

Lethbridge, Dona J.
    Promoting effective contraceptive use / Dona J. Lethbridge,
Kathleen M. Hanna.
      p.   cm.
    Includes bibliographical references and index.
    ISBN 0-8261-7840-5
    1. Contraception.   2. Birth control.   I. Hanna, Kathleen M.
II. Title
RG136.L395   1997
613.9'4—dc21   96-46782
                                               CIP

Printed in the United States of America

This book is in memory of my mother, Jean Lethbridge, whom I miss very much, and who gave me strength of will and commitment to my work; and for my three sisters whom I love dearly, Carol Gray, June Fernquist, and Jo-Anna Gervais.

DJL

This book is dedicated to my parents, John and Helen, who have always had faith in me.

KMH

Contents

List of Tables

ix

List of Figures

Foreword

Promoting Effective Contraceptive Use will contribute significantly to the understanding and successful efforts of health professionals to educate and counsel their clients regarding management of fertility. The authors address the issue of contraceptive use as one of primary concern to women. Moreover, they recognize that fertility management occurs in a complex context: the lives of women and men. The text will enhance health care providers' ability to orient their teaching and counseling to the needs and preferences of clients rather than focusing only on the contraceptive methods and their characteristics, such as effectiveness and ease of use. Consideration of the social, interpersonal, and individual context for choosing and using contraception precedes discussion of education and counseling about specific methods of fertility management. In addition, considerations of specific populations in fertility management are discussed, including culture and ethnicity, socioeconomic status, gender, and age. Examples include the considerations of poor women in accessing contraceptive services, men as partners in contraception, adolescent women as novice contraceptors, and midlife women as uncertain contraceptors, unsure about when fertility ends. Critical analysis of contraceptive data is essential to accurate health education and counseling. Approaches to critical analysis serve as a preface to the discussion of hormonal, barrier, natural family planning, intrauterine devices, and ancient methods, as well as sterilization.

The authors critically examine fertility management from multiple perspectives—from the social to the individual—they challenge professionals providing health education and counseling to consider contraception within a broader context than the clinic. This text will be an outstanding companion to those volumes focusing on contraceptive methods and will bring a novel perspective to delivery of fertility management services.

NANCY FUGATE WOODS, PhD, RN, FAAN
Director, Center for Women's Health Research
University of Washington

Contributors

Monica E. Jarrett, PhD, RN, is research associate professor in the Department of Biobehavioral Nursing and Health Systems at the University of Washington in Seattle. Her research focuses on the menstrual cycle and physiological changes during midlife in women.

Dianna Lee Spies Sorenson, PhD, RN is associate professor in the College of Nursing at South Dakota State University. Her research focuses on women's developmental processes with emphasis on childbearing.

Joyce E. White, Dr PH, RN, RNP, is a Family Nurse Practitioner. She coordinates the Family Nurse Practitioner Program at Slippery Rock University.

Acknowledgments

We would like to thank our dear friend and colleague, Dr. Monica Jarrett, for introducing us and for her valued friendship to us both. We also acknowledge our contributors for their enthusiasm, willingness to share their knowledge, and commitment to the area of fertility management. And, we are most grateful to Rozella Coggin for her excellent work with our tables and typescript, as well as her unfailing good humor and support.

In addition, Dona would like to gratefully acknowledge Dr. Nancy Fugate Woods, her postdoctoral sponsor for study in women's health research. During that experience, Dr. Woods was a role model for scholarship that was diligent, rigorous, and always respectful and oriented to women and their needs. The grants provided by the now National Institute for Nursing Research funding the postdoctoral scholarship and subsequently the Center for Women's Health Research at the University of Washington, were responsible for Dona's study, research, and earlier writings on issues related to women's health and fertility management.

Finally, Dona is forever grateful for the love and support of Ethan Scarl, and Austen and Ben Lethbridge-Scarl. Kathy is grateful for the patience and support of family and friends while she was involved (and sometimes overwhelmed) in this endeavor.

Acknowledgments

Introduction

There have been a myriad of studies on contraceptive use, most of them aimed at understanding why women do not use contraception more effectively to prevent unwanted pregnancy. There has been less recognition of the importance and impact of fertility management on women's and men's lives, their personal development and identity; the many relationships that nourish and support them and for which they are responsible; and the worlds that they build and maintain for themselves and their families. Family planning programs tend to be more concerned with the welfare of society as a whole than with the well-being of an individual woman or man. Though China's one-child policy is an extreme example, even industrialized countries have a vested interest in eliminating the financial burden of unwanted children, preventing induced abortions, and reducing family size.

Women and men manage their fertility within a variety of contexts. These are their personal needs, goals, and values; their interpersonal relationships; and the social norms and cultures within which they live. We have organized this book to include discussion and recognition of the influence of each of these. In addition, we consider the contraceptive context, the methods available to women and men, with their varying physiological mechanisms, effectiveness and failure rates, side effects, and contraindications; and the health care system and providers. It is this context that provides women and men the means, limited though they may be, to manage their fertility as best they can.

This book is founded on the perspective that contraceptive use is an issue of primary concern, especially to women. This book focuses on the complexity of women's and men's experience with contraception, and how it affects their lives as a whole. Fertility management is an essential component of well-being. The use of a contraceptive method that is uncomfortable can affect women's lives, not only through the possibility of irregular use and unwanted pregnancies, but through decreasing the quality of their lives throughout the childbearing years.

This book is written for nurses, physicians, family planning counselors, and other health care providers who are able to give the time to women and men, so that they may make the best contraceptive choice possible, and address the possible barriers and difficulties with its use. All health care providers, whatever their discipline and profession, have the responsibility to address the unique perspectives of clients and the complexity of their experience with contraception, and to achieve their childbearing goals in harmony with the many aspects of their lives. The role of the health care provider is to facilitate women's and men's negotiation with the myriad aspects of choosing and using contraception. The health care provider must educate as well as counsel the client. Education provides the client with information she or he needs to make an informed choice, whereas in counseling, the health care provider helps the client to identify and incorporate perceptions, values, goals, and needs. In addition, health care providers may have specific functions, such as prescribing and monitoring the contraceptive method.

This book is written from a specific perspective for addressing women and men who choose and use contraception. One aspect is recognition of the women's and men's personal experiences, needs, and goals. Based on their experiences, women and men have perceptions of benefits and barriers to any contraceptive method and various levels of ability to solve their contraceptive problems. The second is recognizing women's and men's self-determination or ability for self-care in fertility management, as well as other aspects of their lives. The third is recognition of the value of the health care provider and women and men participating together to manage conception control in the very constrained environment of the health care system. It also recognizes the limited role that health care providers truly have in women's and men's conduct of their lives, and that many must live with very limited support from any health care provider at all. Finally, this book is focused on the use of contraception or a priori methods to prevent conception, rather than fertility management methods such as abortion, the morning-after pill, and so on.

This book can be used as a complement to *Contraceptive Technology* by Hatcher and colleagues. *Contraceptive Technology* emphasizes management of contraceptive methods, whereas our book emphasizes management of men's and women's fertility within the context of their complex lives. This book provides some of the same information as *Contraceptive Technology* with the intent that health care providers can use this information as a reference on contraceptive methods while working with their clients. This book is not intended to replace *Contraceptive Technology,* but to provide health care providers with additional insights into men's and women's experience with contraceptive management. With this perspective, one hopes that health care providers will be able to promote independence, informed choices, and appropriate contraceptive techniques that match individuals' and couples' needs, preferences, and expectations. A final caveat must be mentioned: at the time this book went to press, data from the most recent National Survey of Family Growth, presenting national data on contraceptive use and patterns of pregnancy and birth, were not yet available. Thus, survey statistics that are taken from this source are from the 1988 study.

The book is organized within three major themes presented as units. The first provides a framework for considering the contexts in which self-care must occur. Chapter 1 provides the social context that affects the availability of resources for contraceptive choice and use. Chapter 2 provides a description of women and men's experience of contraception within their interpersonal relationships and the health care system. Chapter 3 discusses women's and men's individual decision making or problem solving around a choice of contraception and strategies to facilitate adherence. Within Part Two, Chapters 4 through 7 describe the influence of culture and class, the experiences of females—adolescents, young adults, and midlife women—as well as the special situations of males. In Part Three, Chapters 8 through 14 provide information on various contraceptive methods, organized to focus on the effect of their mechanism of action and use on women and men's physiological, emotional, cognitive, and social well-being.

DONA J. LETHBRIDGE, PHD, RN
KATHLEEN M. HANNA, PHD, RN

PART ONE

Contexts for Choosing and Using Contraception

The chapters in Part One provide an overview of the social, interpersonal, and individual contexts for choosing and using contraception. The first chapter discusses the boundaries and strictures placed by society on contraception, fertility regulation, and childbearing, as well as providing a discussion of societal constraints on resources and contraceptive availability. Chapter 2 describes women's experiences with choosing and using contraception in terms of their feelings about pregnancy, their relationships with their partners, and their negotiations with the health care system. It provides a comprehensive guide for aiding identification and discussion of benefits and barriers to various contraceptive techniques and behaviors. Chapter 3 provides a framework for a strategy to help women and men with their contraceptive decision making. With more deliberative decision making, they will adhere better to their contraceptive choice.

The Social Context for Contraceptive Choice and Use

Dianna Lee Spies Sorenson

A
lthough contraceptive methods have been used for thousands of years, discussion about contraception and contraceptive methods is complex, confusing, and controversial. This chapter addresses issues related to the meaning of contraception, cultural views, reasons for contraceptive use, knowledge, decision-making skills, and access to contraceptive services.

THE MEANING OF CONTRACEPTION

Part of the confusion about contraception stems from conceptual blurring. In essence, there is no singular definition of contraception, and concepts related to contraception are synonymously interchanged. This confusion affects how contraceptive methods are determined, procured, and used.

DEFINITIONAL CONFUSION

The meaning of contraception sometimes differs between the general public's and health professionals' definitions. For example, the dictionary defines contraception as the intentional prevention of fertilization (Guralnik, 1974). Professional definitions, however, usually indicate that contraception is the intentional prevention of fertilization or implantation. The difference between definitions becomes significant when ethically laden questions like, "When does life begin?" are asked.

Even when a singular definition is ascribed, many questions arise during operationalization. For example, can abstinence be considered a contraceptive method since there is no ejaculation, thus no possibility for sperm and ovum union? One could then raise the question, can walking (since coitus would be impossible) be prescribed as a contraceptive method? Is interference with a fertilized ovum's implantation a contraceptive method or an abortive method? Should female circumcision (which includes the removal of the clitoris and partial suturing of the labia) be marketed as a surgical contraceptive method as are tubal occlusion and vasectomy? These questions and others serve as bases for public policy debate.

INTERCHANGEABILITY OF TERMS

Although not a synonym, the term "contraception" is interchangeably substituted with "birth control." Birth control is a broad term that refers to the intentional prevention of live births. Where the overall desired outcome of contraceptive use is the prevention of live births, technically, the term contraception is limited to prevention of fertilization or implantation, which precludes live births. Although contraception can be considered one type of birth control, birth control is not limited to contraception. The interchange of terms perpetuates confusion about what contraception is, and what it isn't.

Another source of confusion related to the interchange of terms is an inherent myth perpetuated by the literal meaning of the term "birth control," which implies that births can be absolutely and perfectly regulated with a guaranteed black and white outcome that is, a baby was or was not born. When the term birth control is synonymously interchanged with contraception, people are lured to believe that they can "control" fertility through contraceptive methods. Adolescents are particularly susceptible to this lure, because of their developmental predisposition to perceive control, from a concrete cognition, as absolute (Roth, 1993). Unfortunately, contraception is not absolute, it is far from perfect, and offers no guaranteed outcome (Neinstein & Katz, 1986; Pollack, 1992).

CULTURAL VIEW

Another issue that introduces confusion and controversy about contraception is cultural view. Fertility regulation is clearly tied to social beliefs, attitudes, and values, which in turn influence access to education and services (Severy, Thapa, Askew, & Glor, 1993). International comparisons between the United States and similar western European countries show little difference in rates of sexual activity. However, an important distinction is that European countries have lower pregnancy, abortion, and birth rates than the United States (Department of International Economic and Social Affairs, 1988). Lower pregnancy rates among the European countries are attributed to the normative acceptance and accessibility of reproductive health services.

These international statistics challenge the mores of mainstream U.S. culture. Frustration with sexual activity among adolescent, indigent, unmarried, and homosexual populations is and has been the focus of public attention with little regard to the health needs of the sexually active (Roth, 1993). Confusion about contraception is perpetuated by U.S. cultural attitudes and values that reflect anxiety and fear about sexual activity, as well as the belief that sexual activity should be limited to select groups (Frost, 1994; Laumann, Michael, & Gagnon, 1994). The nucleus of debate and controversy over contraception innately reflects centuries of social and religious mores about sexual activity (Woodward, 1994).

Debate

A three-sided debate exists. Within the first side of the debate, contraception is a problem because sexual activity is a fundamental requisite. Hence, the first side of the debate interprets the need for contraception outside of marriage to be intrinsically immoral. The oppositional resolve is to eliminate so-called illegitimate sexual activity by abolishing contraception (Laumann et al., 1994). According to this view, acknowledgment and/or promotion of contraceptive methods is a *legitimization* of sexual activity that culture attempts to limit (Newcomer & Baldwin, 1992).

The second side of the debate argues that acknowledgment of a need for contraception is based on an awareness of sexual activity, but not necessarily an *acceptance or countenance* of sexual activity (Senderowitz, 1992). According to the supporting debate, the prevention of pregnancy and concomitant health problems are issues that can and must be solved, because the perils of disease acquisition and premature parenthood are too high for the individual and society. Contraceptive methods are not viewed as a "cure" for sexual activity, but rather contraceptive methods are valued for their ability to prevent premature pregnancy and protect against sexually transmitted diseases.

The third side of the debate maintains that where abstinence is preferred, contraceptive methods are permissible if they are "natural." Natural contraceptive methods are based on fertility awareness alone without the use of mechanical, chemical, or hormonal methods. According to this moderate perspective, natural family planning avoids side effects encountered by mechanical and chemical contraceptives, promotes conjugal decision making, and respects human life and dignity (Hilgers, 1991).

This three-sided debate does not occur within a vacuum. Debate inextricably includes such long-standing issues as fundamental rights of women to bear children, devaluation of women's reproductive capacity, population overgrowth, religious and moral rules about restricted sexual activity, rights to sexual expression, women's health and status, sex education, and right to life (Abernathy, 1993; Cates, Stewart, & Trussell, 1992; Newcomer & Baldwin, 1992; Pollack, 1992; Rosenberg & Gollub, 1992; Ryder, 1993; Santelli & Beilenson, 1992; Senderowitz, 1992). These high-visibility issues are often used as politicized tools to influence public policy that in turn affects education and access to contraceptive methods (Laumann et al., 1994).

USE OF CONTRACEPTION OTHER THAN PREGNANCY PREVENTION

Although contraceptive methods originally were designed to prevent pregnancy, some contraceptive methods possess documented health-related benefits that have implications beyond the goal of pregnancy prevention. Questions are raised about the degree to which contraceptive and noncontraceptive uses can be considered independent of each other. Because most of the need for noncontraceptive use of contraceptive methods arises from sexual activity and all contraceptive methods directly affect fertility, separation is somewhat artificial. Hence, the overt promotion of specific noncontraceptive use of contraceptive methods in response to sexually transmitted disease (STD) has activated many issues and has added to the growing confusion about contraception.

NON-STD USES

Oral contraceptives (OC) have noncontraceptive applications that offer protection from hormonally related disease and symptomatology. Noncontraceptive uses of OCs include the treatment and/or prevention of dysmenorrhea, benign breast disease, functional ovarian cysts, iron-deficiency anemia, early peri-menopausal symptoms, and endometrial and ovarian cancer (Mishell, Davajan, & Lobo, 1991). However, the majority of women are unaware of the noncontraceptive benefits of oral contraceptives and rarely consider these as pregnancy prevention is the primary reason for selection (Pollack, 1992).

SEXUALLY TRANSMITTED DISEASE

Combined barrier and spermicidal contraceptive methods have been examined for their actual and potential effectiveness to control the contraction and spread of STDs such as gonorrhea, syphilis, genital herpes, venereal warts, hepatitis B, cytomegalovirus trichomoniasis, and more recently, human papilloma virus (HPV) (Rosenberg & Gollub, 1992; Winikoff & Wymelenberg, 1992). However, highly publicized attempts to promote the disease preventative feature of contraceptives did not arise until the sexually transmitted human immunodeficiency virus (HIV) and subsequent acquired immunodeficiency syndrome (AIDS) epidemic became foci of national notoriety (Laumann et al., 1994; Rosenberg & Gollub, 1992; Tucker & Cheng, 1991).

Prevalence statistics highlight ethical dilemmas and the need for further research (Mosher, 1990; U.S. Department of Health and Human Services, 1992). Despite the highly publicized and promoted use of barrier and spermicidal contraceptives to control AIDS transmission among American youth, statistics indicate sexually transmitted diseases remain highest among adolescents (Bell & Holmes, 1984).

In response to the prevalence statistics, several states created legislation that mandates school responsibility for sexuality education, especially that which addresses AIDS and its prevention. Related to these mandates, discussion of abstinence, barrier and spermicidal methods of contraception and, in some situations, the open distribution of condoms have ignited new controversy in the ongoing disputation over sex education in schools (Glassgow, 1992).

Without scientific evidence, opponents of school-based educational programs charge that sex education programs encourage adolescents to engage in sexual activity (Santelli & Beilenson, 1992). However, little evidence exists to indicate that adolescents decrease sexual activity as a result of school health programs, either. Studies indicate that what education *does* do is increase the knowledge and use of contraceptive methods and reduce high-risk behaviors among select sexually active adolescents (Dawson, 1986; Marsiglio & Mott, 1986; Strunin & Hingson, 1987). Furthermore, education mitigates perceived drawbacks that decrease adherence to contraceptive use, such as forethought/advanced planning, precision in application, consistency of use, level of convenience, and motivation (Pollack, 1992; Roth, 1993; Santelli & Belilenson, 1992; Szarewski, 1993; Winikoff & Wymelenberg, 1992).

In this era of health care reform, the public has raised the ethical question: Should national resources be used to publicly promote the use of contraceptive methods for the prevention of STDs when compliance and method effectiveness are not established? To address this question, future research needs to identify the specific determinants of contraceptive use and effectiveness among diverse populations (Santilli & Belilenson, 1992).

KNOWLEDGE, DEVELOPMENTAL DECISION MAKING, AND AVAILABILITY

Contraceptive methods are universally discussed from adult models that have been translated to adolescents. Although chronological age is often used to demarcate the onset of adulthood, developmentally a number of biological and contextual influences need to be considered. Due to the lowered age of menarche and truncated economic capability, some have expanded the adolescent phase of development to include the ages 11 to 25 (Senderowitz, 1992). Whereas biologically, the majority of sexually active adolescents are fecundate "adults," major cognitive differences exist between adolescents and their adult counterparts. Unrecognized differences between adults and adolescents add to the confusion and controversy about contraception.

DIFFERENCES BETWEEN ADOLESCENTS AND ADULTS

Developmental differences between adolescents and adults can be described within the total population of contraceptive knowledge, decisional skills, and access. For this discussion, the population of contraceptive knowledge, decisional skills, and access are conceptualized as a normal statistical distribution curve. The continuum on which the distribution is established ranges from low to high levels of competency. Within early adolescence, knowledge about contraceptive methods exceeds both decisional skills and access to contraceptive methods. In contrast, adults' knowledge, decisional skills, and access distributions are reversed, and more closely approximate the total population curve than do adolescents. Adults have high access to contraceptive methods, and a mature basis for decision-making skills. Yet, in relationship to access and skills, adults may not have acquired proportionate knowledge about contraceptive methods.

KNOWLEDGE

Although recent educational efforts have improved, ignorance about contraceptive methods persists (Senderowitz, 1992). Both adolescents and adults have documented educational needs related to contraception.

Adolescents

Adolescents have little knowledge about contraceptive methods in relationship to the gestalt of knowledge availability. Insufficient or inaccurate knowledge about anatomy and reproductive physiology, including the menstrual cycle and fertility, contribute to risk-taking behaviors because adolescents cannot make an informed choice or appropriately utilize contraceptive methods (Roth, 1993).

To compound these knowledge deficits, adolescents are caught in a cultural double bind that projects the paradoxical message: "sex for young people is dirty, wrong, immoral, irresponsible, dangerous and unhealthy while a barrage of sexual messages and provocation from the media, advertising, fashions and popular culture generally tell young people that it is exciting, glamorous, beautiful and the key to popularity and happiness" (Senderowitz, 1992, p. 210). To be effective, education programs must acknowledge and clearly translate this double-bind and articulate behavioral goals at a developmentally appropriate level (Santelli & Beilenson, 1992). Through the benefit of developmentally appropriate education, socialization, and experience, adolescents' decisional skills related to contraceptive choices can develop to their inherent capacity.

Adults

In contrast to adolescents, adults have the cognitive capacity to acquire more contraceptive knowledge than their adolescent counterparts. Unfortunately, adults often have little more knowledge than adolescents because the only formal sexuality and contraceptive education many receive is through high school education programs (Roth, 1993).

This lack of basic knowledge is a barrier that limits discussion with health care professionals (Roth, 1993). Health care professionals, the primary contraceptive information source for adults, do not always offer a full repertoire of alternatives, nor the supportive education required for successful application (Freda, 1994; Swanson & Corbin, 1983).

Implications

If contraceptive methods and their applications are not recognized and understood, both adults and adolescents are forced to choose among the methods known to them. However, known methods may or may not meet their individual needs. Methods perceived to have undesirable side effects or are expensive, inconvenient, uncomfortable, or overtly obtrusive will not be consistently utilized, if at all (Lethbridge, 1991; Pollack, 1993; Szarewski, 1993). Contraceptive methods will continue to be underutilized if people are not educated about a variety of contraceptive methods and allowed to "customize" those methods to their individual needs.

DECISIONAL SKILLS

A detailed discussion of the differences between adult and adolescent cognitive development and capacity for abstract knowledge acquisition is provided in Chapter 3.

AVAILABILITY

The availability of contraceptive methods embodies a number of barriers. Ineligibility for public assistance combined with prolonged economic dependency on parents and guardians, as well as contraceptive costs, access and the need for anonymity are important barriers to contraceptive availability.

Financial Barriers

Although most prescriptive contraception methods are currently covered by private insurance, one in three women obtain contraceptive methods through subsidized family planning clinics (Henshaw & Torres, 1994).

In general, impoverished women are able to obtain assistance from two federal programs: Medicaid and Title X. Medicaid, a joint federal–state program established through Title XIX of the Social Security Act, provides support for 83% of family planning services budgets. Medicaid reimburses states for 90% of their contraceptive expenditures for eligible low-income women (Kaeser, 1994).

Title X of the Public Health Services Act, a federal program devoted to family planning services for low-income women, provides more than 20% of the budget for family planning clinics (Henshaw & Torres, 1994). To qualify for free services, women must be at or below 100% of the poverty level; sliding scale payments are offered to women who fall between 100% and 250% of the poverty level (Frost, 1994). Furthermore, eligible adolescents can receive these free services without parental consent at clinics that receive Title X funding (Office of the Federal Register, 1988).

Publicly assisted programs that provide services and financial support for contraception have an uncertain fate, as they are subject to national and local economic cutbacks, public policy, and legislation (Henshaw & Torres, 1994). Bound to the abortion and right-to-life debate, legislation designed to limit abortive services may have direct and/or indirect effects on access to contraceptive methods (Laumann et al., 1994). Therefore, the financially dependent may face further contraceptive choice restrictions in the future.

Even now with the current existence of federal, state, and local assistance programs, many low-income women are ineligible for assistance programs. Federally subsidized care for disadvantaged women is not guaranteed, since agencies markedly differ in the types of contraceptive methods offered, criteria for eligibility, and continuity of care. Disadvantaged women are often unable to find clinics that provide minimal-cost services, because many long-term contraceptive methods are prohibitively expensive, even when sliding-scale payments are accepted.

Harvey's (1994) study indicated that there is a clear negative correlation between condom prices and subsequent sales within social marketing programs. He concluded that "price elasticity decreases at the lowest end of the income scale" (Harvey, 1994, p. 57). Thus, among low-income groups and financially dependent adolescents, even an increase of pennies in cost can become a barrier to contraceptive use.

Over-the-counter contraceptive methods that do not require medical evaluation and prescription are less costly, but are also less reliable than prescriptive methods. Contraceptives have a wide range of affordability. Examples, although not an exhaustive list, of the cost of contraceptives are listed in Table 1.1. Costs range from $3 per dozen for condoms and $7 for spermicidal jellies, to over $600 for intrauterine devices, $365 for a 5-year subcutaneous implant device (not including insertion and removal costs), and $45 per month for oral contraceptives (Kaeser, 1994; Winikoff et al., 1992).

Access

Service appointment schedules that conflict with school and working hours restrict access and limit the choice of contraceptive methods. Access to contraceptive services is further restricted due to clinic overcrowding and service provision delays (Moore, 1987).

TABLE 1.1. Examples of Contraceptives' Average Direct and Indirect Costs

Contraceptive	Direct costs	Indirect costs

Condom
  Latex
  Skin
	$3.00 to $18.00 per dozen
	$2.00 each to $30.00 per dozen	

Diaphragm	$12.00 to $25.00 each (multiuse)	Medical examination Lab work Diaphragm fitting Must be used with spermicide

Spermicide
  Creams and jellies
 	
  Vaginal suppositories
  Film
	$7.00 to $11.00 per 3.8 oz. tube (11 applications)
	$0.50 to $0.75 each
	$8.00 per dozen	

Cervical cap	$30.00 to $40.00 (multiuse)	Medical examination Cervical cap fitting Must be used with spermicide
Hormonal Combined	$12.00 to $30.00 per month (approximately $220.00 per year to $225.00 per year)	Annual medical exam Lab work
Progestin only	$25.00 to $45.00 per month (approximately $325.00 to $585.00 per year)	Annual medical exam Lab work
Norplant	$350.00 (if used all 5 years total direct and indirect costs average $100.00 per year)	Physical examination Insertion and removal
Intrauterine devices	$100 and up (8 years of protection)	Physical examination Counseling Follow-up visits Lab work Insertion and removal Prophylactic and analgesics and antibiotics

Source: Winikoff, B., & Wymelenberg, S. (1992).

On-site clinics that include reproductive services have eliminated access barriers related to transportation and clinic operating hours (Kirby, Wazak, & Ziegler, 1991; Zabin et al., 1986). Furthermore, availability and use of a variety of contraceptive methods, and, to a small extent, delayed onset of first coitus are documented benefits of on-site clinics. However, on-site services have been limited to inner-city schools and large corporate businesses, and are highly susceptible to elimination due to budgetary constraints.

Anonymity

Contraceptive service acquisition and contraceptive procurement are often clandestine activities among unmarried and adolescent populations due to social stigmatization. Many unimpoverished adolescents cannot access medically prescribed contraceptives if they have not communicated their sexual activity to their guardians (Henshaw & Torres, 1994). The fear of others (especially parents) knowing about contraceptive use is a major deterrent to contraceptive acquisition and use (Senderowitz, 1992).

Furthermore, anecdotal accounts and case study reports of incentives for contraceptive use, coercion, and inappropriate targeting of select populations to receive contraceptive modalities have escalated public fears about governmentally sponsored contraceptive programs (Frost, 1994). Within an era of informatics and regionalization of health care systems, where anyone related to the health care field will potentially be able to access personal health information, governmental involvement may continue to be misinterpreted.

CONCLUSIONS

Considerable speculation has been and will continue to be made about the philosophical, ethical, and public policy positions of the future (Freda, 1994; Frost, 1994; Henshaw & Torres, 1994; Kaeser, 1994; Klerman, 1994; Rosoff, 1994). To address these positions, the meaning of contraception, cultural view, reason for contraceptive use, knowledge, decision-making skills, and access to contraceptive services will need continued consideration, interpretation, and justification. Clarification of these underlying issues and a clear research agenda are imperative to address the health care needs of all Americans.

REFERENCES

Abernathy, V. (1993). The world's women: Fighting a battle, losing the war. *Journal of Women's Health, 2*(1), 7–16.

Bell, T. A., & Holmes, K. K. (1984). Age-specific risks of syphilis gonor-rhea, and hospitalized pelvic inflammatory disease in sexually experienced United States women. *Sexually Transmitted Diseases, 11,* 291–295.

Cates, W., Stewart, F. H., & Trussell, J. (1992). Commentary: The quest for women's prophylactic methods—hopes vs. science. *American Journal of Public Health, 82*(11), 1279–1482.

Dawson, D. A. (1986). The effects of sex education on adolescent behav-ior. *Family Planning Perspectives, 18,* 162–170.

Department of International Economic and Social Affairs. (1988). *Adolescent reproductive behavior: Evidence from developed coun-tries,* Vol. 1. New York: United Nations Population Studies, 109.

Freda, M. C. (1994). Childbearing, reproductive control, aging women, and health care: The projected ethical debates. *Journal of Obstetric, Gynecologic and Neonatal Nursing, 23*(2), 144–151.

Frost, J. J. (1994). The availability and accessibility of the contracep-tive implant from family planning agencies in the United States, 1991–1992. *Family Planning Perspectives, 26*(1), 4–10.

Glassgow, E. (1992). Where do we go from here? *South Dakota Family Newsletter, 92*(3), 1–4.

Guralnik, D. B. (ed.) (1974). *Webster's new world dictionary of the Ameri-can language.* New York: William Collins World Publishing.

Harvey, P. D. (1994). The impact of condom prices on sales in social marketing programs. *Studies in Family Planning, 25*(1), 52–58.

Henshaw, S. K., & Torres, A. (1994). Family planning agencies: Services, policies and funding. *Family Planning Perspectives, 26*(2), 52–59.

Hilgers, T. W. (1991). *The medical applications of natural family plan-ning.* Omaha, NE: Pope Paul VI Institute Press.

Kaeser, L. (1994). Public funding and policies for provision of the con-traceptive implant, fiscal year 1992. *Family Planning Perspectives, 26*(1), 11–16.

Klerman, L. V. (1994). Perinatal health care policy: How it will affect the family in the 21st century. *Journal of Obstetric, Gynecologic and Neonatal Nursing, 23*(2), 124–128.

Laumann, E. O., Michael, R. T., & Gagnon, J. H. (1994). A political history of the national sex survey of adults. *Family Planning Perspectives, 26*(1), 34–38.

Lethbridge, D. J. (1991). Women's experience with contraception:

Towards a theory of contraceptive self-care. *Nursing Research, 40,* 276–280.

Marsiglio, W., & Mott, F. L. (1986). The impact of sex education on sexual activity, contraceptive use and premarital pregnancy among American teenagers. *Family Planning Perspectives, 18,* 151–162.

Mishell, D. R., Davajan, V., & Lobo, R. A. (eds.) (1991). I*nfertility, contraception, and reproductive endocrinology.* Boston: Blackwell Scientific Publications.

Moore, M. L. (1987). Appointments for adolescent pregnancy and family planning: The effects of delays in providing services. *Public Health Nursing, 4*(1), 43–47.

Mosher, W. D. (1990). Contraceptive practice in the United States, 1982–1988. *Family Planning Perspectives, 22,* 198–205.

Neinstein, L. S., & Katz, B. (1986). *Contraception and chronic illness: A clinician's sourcebook.* Atlanta, GA: American Health Consultants.

Newcomer, S., & Baldwin, W. (1992). Demographics of adolescent sexual behavior, contraception, pregnancy, and STDs. *Journal of School Health, 62*(7), 265–327.

Office of the Federal Register. (1988). *Code of federal regulations* (Part 42 of a codification of documents of general applicability and future effect). Washington, DC: U.S. Government Printing Office.

Pollack, A. E. (1992). Teen contraception in the 1990s. *Journal of School Health, 62*(7), 288–293.

Rosenberg, M. J., & Gollub, E. L. (1992). Commentary: Methods women can use that may prevent sexually transmitted disease, including HIV. *American Journal of Public Health, 82*(11), 1473–1478.

Rosoff, J. I. (1994). The Clinton health plan: What does it do for reproductive health services? *Family Planning Perspectives, 26*(1), 39–41.

Roth, B. (1993). Fertility awareness as a component of sexuality education. *Nurse Practitioner, 18*(3), 40–54.

Ryder, R. E. (1993). "Natural family planning": Effective birth control supported by the Catholic church. *British Medical Journal, 307,* 723–725.

Santelli, J. S., & Beilenson, P. (1992). Risk factors for adolescent sexual behavior, fertility, and sexually transmitted diseases. *Journal of School Health, 62*(7), 271–279.

Senderowitz, J. (1992). Are adolescents good candidates for RU 486 as an abortion method? *Law, Medicine & Health Care, 20*(3), 209–214.

Severy, L. J., Thapa, S., Askew, I., & Glor, J. (1993). Menstrual experiences and beliefs: A multicountry study of relationships with fertility and fertility regulating methods. *Women & Health, 20*(2), 1–20.

Strunin, L., & Hingson, R. (1987). AIDS and adolescents: Knowledge, beliefs, attitudes, and behaviors. *Pediatrics, 79*(5), 825–828.

Swanson, J. M., & Corbin, J. (1983). The contraceptive context: A model for increasing nursing's involvement in family health. *Maternal-Child Nursing Journal, 12*(3), 169–183.

Szarewski, A. (1993). Recent developments in contraception: I. *Professional Care of Mother and Child, 3*(4), 90–91.

Tucker, V. L., & Cheng, T. C. (1991). AIDS and the adolescent. *Postgraduate Medicine, 89*(3), 49–53.

U.S. Department of Health and Human Services. (1992). Sexual behavior among high school students—United States, 1990. *Morbidity and Mortality Weekly Report, 40*(51 & 52), 885–888.

Winikoff, B., & Wymelenberg, S. (1992). *The contraceptive handbook: A guide to safe and effective choices.* Yonkers, NY: Consumer Reports Books.

Woodward, K. L. (1994). Mixed blessings. *Newsweek, CXXII*(7), 38–41.

Zabin, L. S., Hirsch, M. B., Smith, E. A., Streett, R., & Hardy, J. B. (1986). Evaluation of a pregnancy prevention program for urban teenagers. *Family Planning Perspectives, 118,* 119–126.

The Interpersonal Context: Women's Experience of Choosing and Using Contraception

Dona J. Lethbridge

S exuality and reproduction are naturally and inextricably bound. With each episode of heterosexual sexual intercourse between two fertile individuals, there is the possibility of beginning a new life if the necessary physiological factors converge. Yet, sexual relationships have other rewards—they are some of the most pleasurable and affirming pastimes on earth, possibly to ensure that they occur and the species continues.

Now, however, we live in a world in which there are beginning to be too many offspring. In third-world countries, there are not the resources to feed the burgeoning populations. In western countries, societies in which children are not easily integrated have evolved. With everyone away from the home, with the expense of housing, feeding, clothing, and educating household members, there are few to take care of the children and often too little money to raise them. In the People's Republic of China, couples are limited to one child. In the United States, the family norm is two children. Sexual relationships hold couples together as they jointly operate a household and raise children, but once they have their desired number of offspring, sexuality must be separated from reproduction.

Given the complexity of the physiological connection between sexuality and reproduction, the possibility of thwarting the process is underrated by sexually active couples, and perhaps by health care practitioners as well. It has been somewhat jocularly suggested, though accurately as well, that there are 600 million women of reproductive age in the world. There are 39 trillion acts of intercourse per day, 12,000 ejaculations per second, and 60 million sperm per ejaculation—with a total worldwide sperm release of 720 trillion sperm per second (Collins, 1994). All this sperm and all this sexual activity underlines the great difficulty in keeping the number of resulting pregnancies down to those ones that are planned and desired.

And, even in spite of society's need to control its population growth, and couples' need to limit their number of children, the desire to have children come only when planned is probably not a dominant objective throughout the world (Rainwater, 1960). Only in western culture, and perhaps a segment of middle-class culture at that, is the ideal that children should be intended and specifically planned to arrive at a certain time highly valued. The act of intentionally conceiving a child may be so daunting a responsibility that couples might prefer to have it happen "accidentally." Even in other cultures, where the desire to limit children is prevalent, children may be born as they are naturally and unintentionally conceived, with contraceptive activity beginning after the desired family size is reached (Lethbridge & Wang, 1992).

All of this discussion is in support of the notion that preventing pregnancy is a complex and demanding task. Couples attend to the need for contraception with varying degrees of comfort, diligence, and success. The methods to prevent pregnancy are relatively few—all are discussed in this book—and they vary in effectiveness. They also vary in the side effects and difficulties associated with their use. Couples who definitely do not want to become pregnant may feel restricted to the most effective methods—hormonal contraception, whether pills, injection, or implants; the intrauterine device (IUD); or sterilization. However, these may be medically contraindicated or the side effects may be intolerable for some, or their use may be perceived as untenable.

Various contraceptive methods have side effects that can be frightening and uncomfortable. The birth control pill and the IUD may both change women's menstrual cycles. The diaphragm may cause cystitis; spermicidal agents and condoms may cause vaginitis. Women and men differ in their willingness or ability to accept the side effects and problems of these contraceptive methods. For some, the prevention of pregnancy is worth the discomfort; for others, effectiveness and discomfort are given equal consideration. In in-depth interviews with women about their actual contraceptive behaviors, women occasionally reported methods considered relatively ineffective, such as coitus interruptus (withdrawal), breastfeeding, and douching (discussed as ancient contraceptive methods in Chapter 13), and the calculation of infertile days of the menstrual cycle (see Chapter 12).

A MODEL OF CONTRACEPTIVE SELF-CARE

A description of the efforts women, especially, make to prevent pregnancy within the changing and evolving contexts of their lives was developed through two qualitative research studies, in-depth interviews with 55 women of varying age, ethnicity, socioeconomic status, and childbearing status (Lethbridge, 1991; Jarrett & Lethbridge, 1994). Contraceptive self-care was specified within six processes, not necessarily independent. These were separately identified according to the emphasis placed on them by the women participants, according to the needs they perceived for contraception and the childbearing stage of their lives (see Figure 2.1). As the model is presented, illustrative quotations from women participants are presented to validate and articulate particular themes. This model may be used as a basis for assessment of a woman's and man's contraceptive situation and needs (see Table 2.1). It has also been used as a context for selection of content within this book considered to be most relevant to self care and fertility management.

The model described in Figure 2.1 includes a central process that has been called "Choosing and Using Contraception." This central process is encircled by thematic clusters. The outermost is "Engaging in Sexual Behavior;" the next is "Desiring Pregnancy and Children." Immediately surrounding the process of choosing and using contraception are three thematic clusters called "Forestalling Pregnancy," "Assigning the Burden of Contraception," and "Negotiating Contraceptive Gatekeepers."

"Choosing and Using Contraception" concerns selecting a technique or a behavior from those available that will prevent or delay pregnancy when a woman is heterosexually active. It is composed of three thematic clusters. One is "Finding a Contraceptive Method," which describes the process of surveying the techniques or methods perceived to be available, and choosing one that seems to be satisfactory. One theme, "Choosing from Limited Options," was described as selection of a contraceptive method that was best tolerated from the few available. The choices from which a method may be selected are limited, especially if certain methods cause medical contraindications or are not preferred. As a 20-year-old single woman noted: "I wish they could find another way [contraceptive method] . . . I feel like you have problems with everything and I don't have very many options except not being sexually

TABLE 2.1.   Comprehensive Contraceptive Choice and Use Assessment
Guide for Increasing Self-Care
_____

Name: _____

Address: _____
_____

Telephone: _____
(Confidential? _____)

Sexual Relationship/s

_____ Married or partnered, living together (How long? _____)
_____ Partnered, not living together (How long? _____)
_____ Casual relationships
_____ Other _____

I am thinking of leaving my current relationship in the near future.

_____ Yes
_____ No
_____ Maybe

Number of sexual partners at this time _____

Frequency of sexual intercourse _____ WK/MO/YR

My sexual life is very important to me:
_____ Yes
_____ No
_____ Somewhat

Pregnancy and Children

_____ Number of pregnancies
_____ Number of children born
_____ Number of miscarriages
_____ Number of abortions
_____ Number of children living at home
_____ Number of children desired in the future

My feelings about future children are:
_____ I am sad that I will have no more children.
_____ I am very happy that my childbearing days are behind me.
_____ I look forward to having more children.
_____ I wish I could have more children.
_____ Other

Preventing Pregnancy

How important is it that you do not get pregnant now?
_____ Very important
_____ Somewhat important
_____ It would be alright

TABLE 2.1. *(Continued)*

_____ I must not get pregnant now!

When do you plan another pregnancy? _____ WK/MO/YR
_____ I never want to be pregnant again.

Responsibilities for Contraception

In your relationships, who takes the most responsibility for preventing pregnancy?
_____ I do
_____ My partner/s
_____ Responsibility is equally shared

How do you feel about taking responsibility?
_____ I should take it; I bear the burden of pregnancy
_____ I resent that he has no responsibility
_____ I don't mind, one way or the other

Getting the Contraception I Need

Getting along with the doctor/nurse/clinic staff
My relationship with the health care office I go to for contraception is:
_____ Excellent
_____ Good
_____ Alright, but could be better
_____ Poor
_____ I have no health care office to go to for contraception.

My doctor/nurse respects me and my opinions about my contraceptive needs:
_____ Very much
_____ Somewhat
_____ Occasionally
_____ Never

Only some choices of methods of contraception are available from my health care office because:
_____ My doctor or nurse doesn't prescribe certain methods.
_____ My doctor or nurse doesn't believe in certain methods.
_____ My doctor or nurse doesn't believe I will be able to use certain methods well.
_____ My doctor or nurse is prejudiced against me.
_____ My doctor or nurse doesn't listen to me, so doesn't know what I want or need.
_____ Other

I am limited in the kinds of methods I can use because of others:
_____ My parents finding out
_____ My religion
_____ My partner's opinion
_____ Other

(cont.)

TABLE 2.1.   *(Continued)*

Choosing and Using contraception

Finding a contraceptive method

Which of the following contraceptive methods do you know you could get if you wanted them?

_____ Birth control pills
_____ Three month birth control injections (Depo provera)
_____ Birth control implants (Norplant)
_____ IUD (coil or loop)
_____ Diaphragm and jelly
_____ Cervical cap
_____ Contraceptive foam
_____ Female condom
_____ Male condom
_____ My partner using withdrawal
_____ Natural family planning, fertility awareness, rhythm
_____ None
_____ Other

Of the following methods, which ones would you use?

_____ Birth control pills
_____ Three month birth control injections (Depo provera)
_____ Birth control implants (Norplant)
_____ IUD (coil or loop)
_____ Diaphragm and jelly
_____ Cervical cap
_____ Contraceptive foam
_____ Female condom
_____ Male condom
_____ My partner using withdrawal
_____ Natural family planning, fertility awareness, rhythm
_____ Other
_____ None

What methods have you used in the past?

_____ Birth control pills
_____ Three month birth control injections (Depo provera)
_____ Birth control implants (Norplant)
_____ IUD (coil or loop)
_____ Diaphragm and jelly
_____ Cervical cap
_____ Contraceptive foam
_____ Contraceptive sponges
_____ Female condom
_____ Male condom
_____ My partner using withdrawal

TABLE 2.1. *(Continued)*

_____ Natural family planning, fertility awareness, rhythm
_____ Other
_____ None

What methods that you have used have you liked?
_____ Birth control pills
_____ Three month birth control injections (Depo provera)
_____ Birth control implants (Norplant)
_____ IUD (coil or loop)
_____ Diaphragm and jelly
_____ Cervical cap
_____ Contraceptive foam
_____ Contraceptive sponges
_____ Female condom
_____ Male condom
_____ My partner using withdrawal
_____ Natural family planning, fertility awareness, rhythm
_____ Other
_____ None

Using Contraception

How regularly do you use contraception overall?
_____ I always use it, every time I have intercourse.
_____ I miss a few times, but mostly I use it regularly.
_____ I use it when it is available, but I miss sometimes.
_____ I haven't used it very often.
_____ I have never used it.

What is your style of using contraception?
_____ I have chosen one method and I always use it.
_____ I have changed from one method to another over time.
_____ I mix and match; one day I use one method, one day another.
_____ When I have to, I use "unsafe" methods like withdrawal or douching.
_____ I always know if I am at the time in my menstrual cycle when I can get pregnant.
_____ Other

Use of natural family planning/fertility awareness:
_____ I know what time of the month I am fertile and abstain from sex at those times.
_____ I know what time of the month I am fertile and use a contraceptive method on those days.
_____ I do not know or pay attention to what time of the month I might be fertile.

Knowing when you are fertile:
_____ I know by the calendar, where I am in my menstrual cycle.

(cont.)

TABLE 2.1.   *(Continued)*

_____ I know by watching changes in my cervical mucus.

_____ I know by taking my temperature every day.

_____ I know because I have pain in my abdomen when I ovulate in the middle of the month.

_____ Even though I am nearing menopause, I know I am still fertile because of my personal or family history.

_____ I know I am less fertile because I am older now.

_____ I know I am less fertile because I have had trouble getting pregnant.

_____ Other

_____ I have no idea when I might be fertile.

The times I have not used contraception when I should have:

_____ I was in a sexual situation and I had none.

_____ I couldn't get hold of a method in time and was in a sexual relationship.

_____ I have no idea why I did not use any some of those times.

_____ I was not able to get anything to use.

_____ I felt like I might have liked to get pregnant, even though I knew it wasn't a good idea.

_____ I think I was being self-destructive or trying to get myself in trouble.

_____ My partner did not want us to use anything.

_____ Other

The possibility of abortion:

_____ I would have an abortion if I ever felt I needed to.

_____ I would consider having an abortion, but it would be a very hard decision.

_____ I would consider having an abortion if there was something wrong with the baby.

_____ I would consider having an abortion if my life depended on it.

_____ I would consider having an abortion if I was raped.

_____ I would never have an abortion under any circumstances.

The benefits and costs of contraception:

_____ I have had a lighter menstrual flow with my contraception and been happy about it.

_____ I have had fewer menstrual cramps because of my contraception.

_____ I have had a lighter menstrual flow or no flow, and not liked it.

_____ I have had menstrual spotting or bleeding midmonth.

_____ I have had a heavier flow due to my contraceptive method.

_____ I have gained weight from my contraceptive method.

_____ I have had acne (pimples) from my contraceptive method.

_____ When I have used a contraceptive method, it has made me swell up and/or have sore breasts.

_____ I have had vaginal infections when I used contraception.

_____ I am allergic to some contraceptive methods.

TABLE 2.1. *(Continued)*

_____ I have had bladder infections because of my contraceptive method.
_____ My vaginal area has become painful when I have used a contraceptive method.
_____ Other

I sometimes think that my contraceptive methods might have or may make me infertile:
_____ Yes
_____ No

I sometimes wonder if I have been infertile all along, and not known it:
_____ Yes
_____ No

It is more important that I have a very reliable method of birth control, even if it has side effects:
_____ Yes
_____ No

It is more important that I have a contraceptive method that is safe for me even if it is not as reliable in preventing pregnancy:
_____ Yes
_____ No

I never know if my birth control method is causing me trouble, or if it is just me:
_____ Yes
_____ No

I am so happy to be free from the possibility of pregnancy that I use contraception happily:
_____ Yes
_____ No

Other comments: _____
_____
_____
_____
_____

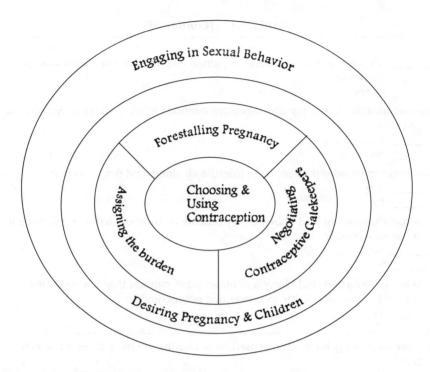

Figure 2.1.   Model for choosing and using contraception.

active which . . . I'm not willing to do right now." Along with a good history and physical examination to identify contraceptive contraindications, strong feelings and preferences about contraception should be
assessed. The other theme was entitled "Celebrating a Good Method,"
described as finding a method that could be used comfortably and regularly. It is the thesis of this book that the method that is most acceptable to a woman and man is the one with the greatest likelihood of
being used regularly and properly. Similarly, sometimes a good method
is hard to find.

The second thematic cluster is "Managing Contraceptive Use," apply-
ing a technique or behavior to prevent pregnancy within a changing
and evolving life situation. The theme "Using Contraception" included
experiences using methods on long-term and short-term bases, often
more than one method at a time, consecutively or sequentially, and on
occasion, in emergency situations, less commonly accepted methods
such as douching. A thorough contraceptive history from the beginning of a woman's or man's sexual initiation is essential. Probing is

often necessary to identify early methods of contraception that might have been less conventional, but were attempts to prevent conception. A contraceptive history will also reveal those methods that were perceived to give difficulty and might not be used regularly or well.

The theme "Calculating Safe Times" described some women's relaxation of contraceptive use during days of the menstrual cycle considered to be infertile. Women who were not using hormonal contraception, an IUD, or sterilization, but who were using coitus-related methods, spoke about the use of the infertile period of their menstrual cycle. This contraceptive behavior is discussed in more detail in Chapter 12 on Natural Family Planning. When midlife women were interviewed about their contraceptive use, and described their sense of waning fertility (Jarrett & Lethbridge, 1994), the title of the theme was changed to the more global "Estimating Fertility," which was described as considering whether, and to what extent, a woman perceived pregnancy possible. This theme, therefore, may occur on a month-to-month basis or be a total summation of the state of fertility. Midlife women used the continued presence of menses, bodily awareness of ovulation, a family history of late pregnancies, a personal history of late pregnancies, and their desire to be fertile as some factors in their estimation of fertility. Other women assumed infertility because of past experiences with pregnancy not occurring, and family history.

The theme "Neglecting Contraception" was described as forgoing any contraceptive behavior or method for an occasional or extended period of time. Occasional or even single lapses were remembered and discussed when they resulted in a pregnancy. It was difficult for women to explain the periods in which they did not use contraception, in spite of attempts to help them to reflect on possible meanings of their actions. Since most contraceptive research takes place to study this very behavior, women's lack of access to the meaning of their behavior suggests that more practical models of intervention might be more fruitful rather than additional attempts at understanding and attempting to change the mechanisms of behavior.

Finally, "Considering the Possibility of Abortion" described women's contingency planning if a pregnancy should occur. The possibility of abortion was described in varying degrees, from a certainty if pregnancy occurred, to perhaps preventable if situational factors permitted another or a child. This theme was more apparent in interviews with midlife women than in interviews with women generally, possibly reflecting the statistic that over 50% of unintended pregnancies in women between the ages of 40 and 44 are terminated through induced abortion (Henshaw, Koonin, & Smith, 1991). A woman's and man's feelings about, and a woman's willingness to undergo abortion should be a part of fertility management assessment. Although there is little evidence to suggest that abortion is used as a contraceptive method, in spite of myths to the contrary, less theoretically effective methods might be considered an option if abortion is available in the case of failure. On the other hand, a woman and man with economic resources and social support might prohibit the use of abortion, but be able to absorb an unintended pregnancy into their lives.

Another thematic cluster was named "Experiencing Contraceptive Costs and Benefits," describing the negative and positive outcomes accrued through using various contraceptive methods and behaviors. It is composed of five themes. One was "Monitoring Body Changes," described as attending to physiological changes related to contraceptive use. Women discussed menstrual cycle changes, such as decreased menstrual flow or menstrual spotting with hormonal techniques, or other physiological changes such as weight gain, acne, edema, breast tenderness, vaginal candidiasis, bladder infections, or genital irritation from spermicidal agents.

Menstrual changes deserve special mention, as feelings about menstruation are often extreme, whether negative or positive. For many women, menses have a negative connotation, and anything that might make their cycles easier to withstand would be welcomed. This might include alleviation of premenstrual symptoms, dysmenorrhea, or menorrhagia. Others relish the regularity of their menses as it suggests that pregnancy has not occurred, regular occurrence denotes health, and is a symbol of womanhood (Chrisler, Johnston, Champagne, & Preston, 1994). In some cultures, menstrual flow represents the release of bodily toxins and is associated with internal cleanliness (see Chapter 7).

Another theme was entitled "Balancing Reliability with Side Effects." Side effects and difficulties were sometimes described as inevitable inconveniences, but sometimes as overwhelming. One woman said, "I worry about effectiveness but I don't use methods that are more effective because I'm worried more about the side effects of those methods."

Versus another who said, "I don't care about side effects; I cannot get pregnant."

"Attributing Side Effects" was described as determining if experienced symptoms were due to the contraceptive method or to factors within the women themselves. As one woman explained, "I've always had a hard time being objective about myself, and I would have crying spells, I was very upset all the time. I saw it happen to my sisters . . . I had never put two and two together until I figured out we were all taking the pill."

"Valuing Sexual Freedom" included enjoying sexual relationships while minimizing the possibility of pregnancy, and "Gaining Other Benefits" were outcomes of contraceptive use that led to an increased feeling of well-being. For example the use of the birth control pill also increased menstrual regularity. Condoms also protect from disease.

It is clear that this central theme of Choosing and Using Contraception relates both to the number of methods and behaviors that are available, on the market, and usable by a specific couple, and the knowledge and awareness, beliefs, and attitudes about contraception a couple bring to their situation. Their tolerance for discomfort is also a factor. This central theme exemplifies the challenge of finding a method that may be used successfully and comfortably by a couple so that their sexual relationship is minimally disrupted by contraceptive needs and the chance of an unwanted pregnancy is minimized.

The contraceptive self-care process of Choosing and Using Contraception in general was elaborated with the experiences of midlife women, since their contraceptive patterns were specific to their greater experience with contraception and changing physiology. Women described previous experiences with cancer and other pathophysiology that limited their contraceptive options as well as changing menstrual patterns that made fertility awareness difficult if not impossible. Most women had experience with many contraceptive methods and had settled on a method that they could use with some satisfaction.

Surrounding the central thematic clusters were more encompassing thematic clusters of Engaging in Sexual Behavior and Desiring Pregnancy and Children. "Engaging in Sexual Behavior" was specifically identified from data from midlife women. It would most likely have been identified from a more general population of women, but many studies of contraceptive use, like the other one reported here, was limited to those women in heterosexual relationships and actively needing contraception. Women's sexual activities, however, may be in flux, in a long-term relationship with sporadic sexual activities, in serial monogamous relationships, or between relationships with any future relationship uncertain.

The nature of sexual relationships was a prevalent issue for midlife women, possibly because often they were changing during this time. Sexual activity ranged from the adoption of sexual abstinence, to lesbian relationships, to a relishing of heterosexual activity as the prospect of pregnancy waned. Some women talked about sexual interest peaking during midcycle and their sadness that, with waning fertility, would come waning sexuality.

There are three themes within this process. They are "Living with Sexual Abstinence," described as a voluntary or involuntary absence of sexual relationships. As one woman poignantly said, "I looked forward to my forties . . . I thought of myself as, "Oh honey, you're going to be foxy and 40, you're going to know so much . . . be more adept sexually . . .' I just don't have anybody to practice this with."

Another theme was named "Continuing Ongoing Sexual Relationships" and described passing through life with a partner of many years, and established sexual patterns and behaviors. The third theme was "Relishing Sexuality" described as an appreciation of sexuality and sexual relationship(s).

Needless to say, sexual partnerships must be assessed. It should not be assumed that a woman is heterosexual, with the possibility of a pregnancy. Nor should monogamy be assumed, even in the case of a marriage. Women who are recently out of a relationship are at risk for unprotected intercourse, since they may have discontinued use of a contraceptive method and then unexpectedly enter into a new relationship. They should be warned of this possibility.

Another encompassing process was "Desiring Pregnancy and Children" and described as feelings about past experiences with pregnancy and childrearing and the loss of the ability to have those experiences or have them again. The two themes were striking in the interviews with women as they age.

"Mourning the Passing of Childrearing" was described as reflecting on childrearing as a stage of life that was positive and important, but was soon to be over. For some women, this took the form of hoping for an (additional) child while it was still possible. An example is a woman who suffered an unwanted and subsequently terminated pregnancy as her first child went off to college. This may also be relevant to women and men as they consider, anticipate, go through, and recover from sterilization (see Chapter 15).

"Celebrating the Closure of Fertility" described women's positive feelings in being done with the possibility of childbearing and the tasks of childrearing. Many opportunities, activities, and freedoms are availed to women and men as their children grow and become more independent. While childbearing and childrearing are among the richest and most profound of life's experiences for many women and men, it happens, earlier or later, that those times are finished and other destinies are revealed. The situation of the midlife woman is described in detail in Chapter 7.

There are three thematic clusters that surround Choosing and Using Contraception that may have a more immediate influence on contraceptive choices and the management of fertility. "Forestalling Pregnancy," the desire to prevent or delay conception, included three themes.

"Fear of Unwanted Pregnancy" described the fear of having a mistimed child or induced abortion, and is consistent with "Valuing Freedom from Childbearing." "Fearing Future Infertility" described the fear of not being able to have a child when desired, either because of preexisting infertility or because of contraceptive methods used. As one woman said, "I always get this really weird feeling—what's going to happen when we decide to have a family and if I cannot conceive . . .. That has always worried me."

The unwarranted fear of side effects of contraception has long been an issue in women's and men's failing to consider or use certain methods (Pipert & Gutmann, 1993). Still, it is important that the benefits of fertility management be recognized. While many women and men may indeed choose to have children unplanned, as they arrive, the disadvantages of mistimed children are onerous. Educational and occupational opportunities are most likely when having children is postponed (Lethbridge, 1990). See Chapter 4 for a more detailed discussion of the influences and consequences of culture and socioeconomic status on fertility management.

Another process influencing "Choosing and Using Contraception" was "Assigning the Burden of Contraceptive Responsibility." One theme, "Bearing the Burden," described women's feeling that contraception was a task that was solely theirs since they bore the brunt of a mistimed pregnancy. Women perceived men as being less upset at the thought of a baby, or less diligent in following through with contraception. Another theme was labeled "Resenting the Burden," begrudging the partner's escape from the inconvenience and effort of contraception, while having the sexual pleasure. However, burden for contraception may be shared with partners. "Sharing the Burden" described allowing partners to take some or all of the responsibility for contraception, because they could be trusted. A woman planning marriage said, "C. even said he wishes they'd have a birth control for men. He would do it—the burden to be the one to worry about it. He never really wanted me to take the pill, because he didn't feel he wanted me to be in the position of taking that kind of a powerful medication." To a lesser extent, women encouraged their partners to participate by paying for contraceptive methods or helping with tasks such as transportation to health care appointments.

Men's participation in fertility management may be culturally specific (see Chapters 4 and 5). It also should be noted that the description in this chapter is derived from women's perceptions—of their own need to take responsibility, and of men's reluctance to do so. Since there are only few methods of contraception that may be used by men and, of these, condoms and withdrawal are considered less reliable in preventing pregnancy, men are limited as to how much direct effect they may have. It goes without saying that men should be included in the fertility management assessment and treatment process. Men's health care should also include fertility management as a standard component.

The final process was "Negotiating the Contraceptive Gatekeepers." This process describes maneuvering among the individuals and agencies that permit or hinder access to contraceptive methods and behaviors. One theme was "Using the Health Care System," working with health care professionals and health care systems to obtain access to those contraceptive methods available only through prescription. This theme is described in Chapter 1. Although some women had established positive relationships with health care providers and received help in obtaining contraception, others see the health care system as responsible for limiting research on new methods, especially those that might be used by men. On an individual level, women are limited in their selection of methods if their health care provider does not prescribe, for example, certain brands of birth control pills or the cervical cap, or does not believe specific methods are appropriate for an individual woman. In one case, a woman who wished to change from an IUD to a diaphragm said, "When I went to get my IUD out, he [the physician] refused and said I would just get pregnant again. So I had to go to another doctor, and she took it out."

A Native American woman, however, described her experience with a publicly funded physician, that verged on coercion. Twenty-one years old and unmarried, she recalled her extreme fear of surgery as she was being wheeled to her second cesarean birth, "It [the choice] wasn't up to me. The doctor just said, I think you ought to have your tubes tied because I don't think you want to have any more kids. . . . So I just said okay." This woman grieved her early sterilization, and at 38, still thought about ways she might have a reversal.

Another theme was entitled "Abiding by Religious Laws or Cultural Norms," in which women described managing contraceptive use to conform to strictures set by social authorities. A 27-year-old married woman using barrier methods said, "I went off the pill because I grew up Catholic, and I always have this terrible, terrible guilt complex about it. . . . How would I tell a priest?"

Finally, a third theme was entitled "Sidestepping the Control of Others," which involved considering and avoiding the wishes of others in choosing and using a contraceptive method. Women discussed the roles of significant others, such as parents and partners, who may also control access to contraception.

STRATEGIES FOR INTERVENTION

Women's and men's health care should include careful attention to fertility management, without assumptions about appropriate methods for individuals, with abiding respect for the difficulty of preventing pregnancy in heterosexual relationships, and with appreciation of the difficulty of managing fertility when there are so few methods and behaviors available even yet, and those fraught with side effects and disadvantages.

Table 2.1 provides a comprehensive guide based on the model for discussion with women and men about their contraceptive use and goals. Although some practitioners use scored instruments to help women and men choose a method (see Hatcher et al., 1994 for an example), it is important to recognize that any one factor, a perception, or objective characteristic, present or in the future, may jeopardize the use of a selected method. This comprehensive guide will highlight areas of conflict or difficulty that should be taken into consideration as contraceptive choice and use is discussed together by provider and clients. Women and men should consider the full array of contraceptive options in terms of their own situations. Careful and thorough assessment of the life situation in all its complexity and uncertainty will make optimum fertility management more of a possibility.

REFERENCES

Chrisler, J. C., Johnston, I. K., Champagne, N. M., & Preston, K. E. (1994). Menstrual joy: The construct and its consequences. *Psychology of Women Quarterly, 18,* 375–387.

Collins, E. B. (1994). *New developments in contraception.* Paper presented to Contraception for the 90s, University of Alabama in Huntsville Clinical Science Center, August 12, 1994.

Hatcher, R. A., Trussell, J., Stewart, F., Stewart, G. K., Knowal, D., Guest, F., Cates, Jr., W., & Policar, M. S. (1994). *Contraceptive Technology,* 16th revised ed. New York: Irvington Publishers.

Henshaw, S. K., Koonin, L. M., & Smith, J. C. (1991). Characteristics of U.S. women having abortions, 1987. *Family Planning Perspectives, 19,* 75–78.

Jarrett, M. E., & Lethbridge, D. J. (1994). Looking forward, looking back: Women's experience with waning fertility during mid-life. *Qualitative Health Research, 4*(4), 370–384.

Lethbridge, D. J. (1990). Use of contraceptives by women of upper socioeconomic status. *Health Care for Women International, 11,* 305–318.

Lethbridge, D. J. (1991). Women's experience with contraception: Towards a theory of contraceptive self-care. *Nursing Research, 40,* 276–280.

Lethbridge, D. J., & Wang, R. (1992). Patterns of contraceptive use of women in Taiwan. *Health Care for Women International, 12,* 431–441.

Peipert, J., & Gutmann, J. (1993). Oral contraceptive risk assessment: A survey of 247 educated women. *Obstetrics & Gynecology, 82,* 112–117.

Rainwater, L. (1960). *And the poor get children.* Chicago: Quadrangle Books.

The Individual Context: Promoting Contraceptive Decision Making and Problem Solving

Kathleen M. Hanna

T his chapter provides a framework for promoting contraceptive
decision making, problem solving, and ultimately, adherence to
contraceptive choice that is based on contraceptive beliefs or perceptions. Elements of contraceptive decision making—contraceptive
attitudes and perceptions—have explained and predicted adolescents'
and adults' contraceptive choice, intentions to use contraceptives, and
actual use of contraceptives (Adler, Kegeles, Irwin, & Wibbeisman,
1990; Condelli, 1986; Ewald & Roberts, 1985; Green, Johnson, & Kaplan,
1992; Jaccard & Becker, 1985; Jemmott & Jemmott, 1990; Morrison,
1989; Orr & Langefeld, 1993; Weisman et al., 1991; Whitley & Schofield,
1985, 1986). The framework also provides a means to communicate
with women and men about contraceptive perceptions to promote
deliberative contraceptive decision making and problem solving. As a
result, potential contraceptive problems may be addressed and greater
contraceptive adherence may occur.

Some of the ideas expressed in this chapter appeared previously in K. M. Hanna (1995).
"The Use of King's Theory of Goal Attainment to Promote Adolescent's Health Behavior,"
from the book ADVANCING KING'S SYSTEMS FRAMEWORK AND THEORY by M. Frey & C.
Sieloff (Eds.), pp. 239–250, copyright © 1995 by Sage. Reprinted by permission of Sage
Publications, Inc. Additional material appeared in K. Hanna (1993). Effect of nurse–client
transaction on female adolescents' oral contraceptive adherence. *IMAGE: Journal of
Nursing Scholarship, 25,* 285–290. Copyrighted material of Sigma Theta Tau International.
Used by permission.

CONTRACEPTIVE PERCEPTIONS

Beliefs or perceptions provide a means to understand behavior. Perceptions reflect an individual's way of organizing and interpreting the world (King, 1981, p. 24). One's view of the world is reflected in perceptions that are subjective (Gibson, 1969; King, 1981). These perceptions are influenced by expectations and needs (Bruner, 1973) and emotions (Nisbett & Ross, 1980). Perceptions are influenced by an individual's interactions with others in one's environment (King, 1981).

Perceptions can be delineated more specifically and one framework for delineating health perceptions is the Health Belief Model (HBM) (Rosenstock, 1966). Perceptions of susceptibility, seriousness, benefits, and barriers constitute a cluster of beliefs within a decision-making process which influences health behaviors. These perceptions have been defined with (1) perceived susceptibility as the subjective risk of contracting the condition, (2) perceived seriousness as the belief about the seriousness of the condition, (3) perceived benefits as the belief about the availability as well as the effectiveness of the health behavior, and (4) perceived barriers as the belief about the negative aspects of the health behavior (Rosenstock, 1966, p. 99–100). Perceived susceptibility and seriousness together are a health threat that provide the readiness for action. Perceived benefits are weighed against perceived barriers in making a decision about the health behavior.

Support is suggested for the HBM (Rosenstock, 1966). A positive relationship between health behaviors and perceived susceptibility, seriousness, and benefits has been reported while a negative relationship has been reported between perceived barriers and health behaviors (Becker, 1976; Becker & Janz, 1985; Haynes, 1976; Janz & Becker, 1984; Mikhail, 1981; Redeker, 1988). The most empirical support exists for the relationship between perceived barriers and health behaviors (Janz & Becker, 1984).

Perceptions of the HBM can be applied to the area of contraception. Those who perceive that they are susceptible to becoming pregnant and that pregnancy and parenthood (the condition) would be serious for them seek contraceptives (readiness for action). Those who perceive more contraceptive benefits than barriers will be more likely to decide to use a contraceptive method (the health behavior).

CONTRACEPTIVE PERCEPTIONS

Adolescents and adults have contraceptive perceptions that may influence their contraceptive behavior. One of the first studies to identify contraceptive perceptions was conducted by Luker (1975) with adolescent and adult females attending an abortion clinic. Perceived contraception barriers were having to acknowledge sexuality to self and others; planning to be sexually active having negative connotations; maintaining contraceptive behavior; obtaining contraceptives; and having biological/medical costs. For delineation of adults' and adolescents' contraceptive perceptions, see Chapters 2, 5, 6, and 7.

Contraceptive perceptions have been reported to influence contraceptive behavior. Intentions to use, as well as actual use of contraceptives, have been associated with: (1) greater perceived susceptibility of pregnancy (Arnett, 1990; Namerow et al., 1987; Tanfer et al., 1993; White, 1984), STDs (Orr & Langefeld, 1993), or HIV (Goodman & Cohall, 1989; Tanfer et al., 1993); (2) greater perceived seriousness of AIDS (Pleck et al., 1993); and (3) greater perceived contraceptive benefits and fewer barriers (Balassone, 1989; Cvetkovich & Grote, 1983; DiClemente et al., 1992; Joffe & Radius, 1993; Leland & Barth, 1992; Lowe & Radius, 1987; Loewenstein & Furstenberg, 1991; Kegeles, Adler, & Irwin, 1989; Maticka-Tyndale, 1991; Scher, Emans, & Grace, 1982; Smith, Beck, & Davies, 1987; Strader & Beaman, 1989; Tanfer & Rosenbaum, 1986; Tanfer et al., 1993; Weisman et al., 1991; Walter et al., 1993).

COGNITIVE FUNCTIONING

Cognitive functioning influences contraceptive perceptions, decision making, and problem solving (Hanna, 1995). The ability for advanced problem solving or reasoning usually develops during adolescence (Piaget, 1972). The same level of cognitive functioning may not be present for all areas of cognitive functioning (Piaget, 1972). Variability does exist with some adolescents and adults not attaining advanced reasoning abilities (Martorano, 1977; Neimark, 1975; Tomlinson-Keasey, 1972; White, 1984). Problem solving in a specific area is dependent upon knowledge (Chi & Glaser, 1980; Hayes-Roth et al., 1981; Langley & Simon, 1981; Larkin et al., 1980) and experience (Newell & Rosenbloom, 1981) specific to that area. Therefore, becoming an expert problem solver in the area of contraception involves acquiring contraceptive knowledge and contraceptive experience.

The importance of cognitive functioning specific to contraception is supported in several studies. General cognitive functioning does influence contraceptive cognitive functioning (Green et al., 1992; Sachs, 1985), but alone does not influence contraceptive use (Graber, 1986; White, 1984). Cognitive functioning specific to an area is needed to influence behavior in that specific area. This is supported in that contraceptive use was associated with contraceptive knowledge (Sachs, 1985) and cognitive functioning specific to contraception (Graber, 1986).

When contraceptive experiences are limited, contraceptive perceptions may be affected by cognitive functioning. With both adolescents or adults, cognitive functioning most likely will not be at an expert level when contraceptive knowledge and experience is limited. Those with limited contraceptive experience may not perceive the consequences of their sexual and contraceptive behavior, that is, perceived susceptibility, seriousness, benefits, and barriers. With the failure to perceive consequences, consideration of the consequences of pregnancy and parenthood and the weighing of perceived contraceptive benefits and barriers is impeded. Further, how to problem solve potential contraceptive problems would not occur. For example, a client who is seeking oral contraceptives for the first time may not perceive that remembering to take the pill at the same time everyday will be difficult, and may not think of ways to remember the pill.

PROMOTING CONTRACEPTIVE
DECISION MAKING/PROBLEM SOLVING

Health care providers have the potential for influencing individuals' perceptions through interactions with them. In nursing, for instance, interpersonal relationships or interactions are central to providing care (King, 1981; Levine, 1971; Orlando, 1972; Patterson & Zderad, 1976; Peplau, 1952; Rubin, 1968). Through interpersonal relationships, health care providers can be influential (Rodin & Janis, 1979). Health behavior has been shown to be influenced by interactions that are individualized (Benfari, Eaker & Stoll, 1981; Neufeld, 1976).

Interactions are delineated as two types: informational and influential communication (Kasch, 1986; Kasch & Knutson, 1985; Kasch & Lisnek, 1984; King, 1981). Informational communication is an interaction that provides information or specific facts. Influential communication is a perceptually based interaction that takes into account the woman or man's subjective perspectives, uniqueness, and individuality (Kasch & Knutson, 1985; Kasch & Lisnek, 1984; King, 1981). Perceptions are assumed to be influenced by influential communication (Kasch & Knutson, 1985; Kasch & Lisnek, 1984; King, 1981). Informational communication is reflected in educational strategies, and influential communication is reflected in counseling strategies.

Findings of studies suggest support for the relationship between health behavior and influential communication—perceptually based interactions. Communication by nurses that was more personal in nature was associated with more personalized communication from patients (Orlando, 1972). Provider and client behaviors that were identified as perceptually based interactions and that led to mutually desired goals were as follows: one member initiated behavior via asking questions or making statements; the opposite member responded; problems were identified and noted; goals were mutually agreed upon by both; means to achieve goals were explored; and the members agreed on ways to achieve the goals (King, 1981).

Findings of studies suggest support for the relationship between contraceptive use and contraceptive care provider and client interactions. Contraceptive use was positively associated with interactions in which providers reported that they did use persuasion with clients (Nathanson & Becker, 1985). A group discussion of perceptions based on the HBM was associated with greater levels of perceived seriousness of pregnancy, parenthood, and contraceptive benefits, and lower levels of perceived contraceptive barriers (Eisen, Zellman, & McAlister, 1985). Personalized interactions that were more than provision of contraceptive information positively influenced contraceptive use (Berger et al., 1987; Danielson et al., 1990; Eisen et al., 1990; Hanna, 1993; Marcy, Brown, & Danielson, 1983; Namerow, Weatherby, & Williams-Kaye, 1989).

STRATEGIES FOR INTERVENTION

Strategies should include provision of information on contraception and fertility (please refer to chapters on specific contraceptive methods for information to provide). Contraceptive use has been associated with knowledge of pregnancy risk and contraception knowledge (Balassone, 1989; Levinson, 1995). However, information alone is not sufficient to affect contraceptive behavior. In reviewing interventions that provide information on sexual matters, knowledge has been increased, but the effect on behavior is inconclusive (Kilman et al., 1981; Voss, 1980). Thus, educational strategies are needed but other strategies are also needed.

To further promote contraceptive use, providers may intervene based on a framework encompassing contraceptive perceptions and provider–client interactions (Hanna, 1995). Contraceptive perceptions may be assessed to provide an understanding of contraceptive behavior. In addition, contraceptive perceptions may be used to promote contraceptive decision making and problem solving. Promotion of contraceptive decision making and problem solving—consideration of their contraceptive perceptions—could affect their contraceptive behavior. Pro-

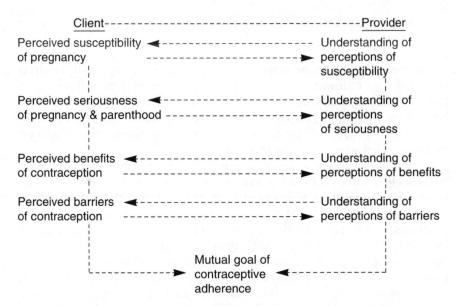

Figure 3.1. Provider and client interaction about contraceptive perceptions to attain a goal of contraceptive adherence.

motion of contraceptive decision making and problem solving may occur through a discussion of contraceptive perceptions between provider and the women and men with whom they work (see Figure 3.1).

AN EXAMPLE: FEMALE ADOLESCENTS AND ORAL CONTRACEPTIVES

Nurse–client interactions based on oral contraceptive perceptions was a nursing strategy tested with a sample of female adolescents seeking oral contraceptives for the first time (Hanna, 1993). The study tested the premise that behavior is influenced by nurse and adolescent interactions that are perceptually based (King, 1981). The purpose of the interaction was to promote the adolescent's oral contraceptive decision making and problem solving, that is, consideration of perceived oral contraceptive benefits and barriers, as well as means to reduce oral contraceptive barriers.

The protocol for the interaction began with the identification of perceived oral contraceptive benefits and barriers. The perceptions were based on research findings of adolescents' perceived oral contraceptive benefits and barriers (Hanna, 1994). In addition, the perceived oral contraceptive barriers were stated specific to the oral contraceptive

TABLE 3.1.   Identification of Perceived Contraceptive Benefits and Barriers

Perceived contraceptive benefits

1. Avoidance of pregnancy out of concern for a friend
2. Avoidance of pregnancy out of concern for parents
3. Avoidance of pregnancy out of concern for partner
4. Avoidance of pregnancy as not ready to be a parent right now or to finish high school or go to college
5. Being responsible
6. Safe and effective in preventing pregnancy

Perceived contraceptive barriers

1. Difficult to get to clinic
2. Difficult to take pills at the same time every day
3. Difficult to keep appointments with the clinic
4. Difficult to call clinic ahead for an appointment
5. Difficult to keep private that one is using pills
6. Using birth control may be against one's beliefs

Source: Hanna (1990).

method and regimen of the clinic. Nurses initiated the discussion of the perceived benefits of oral contraceptives by noting what other young people think are the positive aspects of using oral contraceptives (see Table 3.1). Then perceived oral contraceptives were discussed using the same routine. The interaction was facilitated by using index cards with potential perceived oral contraceptive benefits and barriers statements on each card.

Next in the interaction, adolescents were asked which were positive and which were negative aspects for them, personally. Then barriers that may interfere with oral contraceptive adherence were acknowledged. The goal of preventing pregnancy through use of oral contraceptives was confirmed.

Ways to manage oral contraceptive barriers were explored. Contraceptive use has been noted to be associated with memory strategies (Norris, 1988). Many of the means to manage oral contraceptive barriers revolved around memory strategies such as noting appointments on a calendar, taking a pill at the same time as some other habit such as a meal, and keeping track of the pills in the packet. Inconsistent contraceptive users were reported to forget more frequently than consistent users (Balassone, 1989). Other strategies revolved around privacy (finding a private place to keep pills and to call the clinic) and communication with significant persons (how would you know when to talk with the person, what would you say, and what would the other person say). A frequent reason for contraceptive nonuse was concern about parental reaction to their sexual and contraceptive behavior (Whitley & Schofield, 1985, 1986; Zabin, Stark, & Emerson, 1991). Contraceptive use was greater for those who communicated with partners (Lowenstein & Furstenberg, 1991) and parents about contraceptive matters (Casper, 1990). Finally, oral contraceptive regimen guidelines were reviewed. The following aspects of the protocol include (Hanna, 1990):

I am going to take birth control pills every day at _____ (the same time of day).

I am going to call the clinic for an appointment on _____(date) before I need to refill a prescription; and I am going to remember my appointment with the clinic in 3 months by _____ (memory strategy).

CONCLUSIONS

Women and men hold positive and negative contraceptive perceptions and these contraceptive perceptions influence their contraceptive use. Those who are just beginning to be sexually active and use contraceptives should be considered inexperienced contraceptive decision makers and problem solvers. These individuals may not consider their susceptibility of pregnancy—and seriousness of pregnancy and parenthood—nor perceived contraceptive benefits and barriers. In addition, they may not problem-solve for potential perceived contraceptive barriers.

Promotion of contraceptive decision making and problem solving has the potential to influence adherence to contraceptive choice. Contraceptive information needs to be provided as a beginning basis for contraceptive decision making and problem solving, which then needs to be promoted through perceptually based interactions. With promotion of contraceptive decision making and problem solving, women and men may consider their contraceptive perceptions and ways to address perceived contraceptive barriers. Ultimately, their adherence to their contraceptive choice is promoted through consideration of their contraceptive perceptions.

REFERENCES

Arnett, J. (1990). Contraceptive use, sensation seeking, and adolescent egocentrism. *Journal of Youth and Adolescence, 19,* 171–180.

Balassone, M. (1989). Risk of contraceptive discontinuation among adolescents. *Journal of Adolescent Health Care, 10,* 527–533.

Becker, M. (1976). Sociobehavioral determinants of compliance. In D. Sackett & R. Haynes (eds.), *Compliance with therapeutic regimens* (pp. 40–50). Baltimore: John Hopkins University Press.

Becker, M., & Janz, N. (1985). The Health Belief Model applied to understanding diabetes regimen compliance. *Diabetes Educator, 11,* 41–47.

Benfari, R., Eaker, E., & Stoll, J. (1981). Behavioral interventions and compliance to treatment regimes. *Annual Review of Public Health, 2,* 431–471.

Berger, D., Perez, G., Kyman, W., Perez, L., Garson, J., Menendez, M., Bistriz, J., Blanchard, H., & Dombrowski, C. (1987). Influence of family planning counseling in an adolescent clinic on sexual activity and contraceptive use. *Journal of Adolescent Health Care, 8,* 436–440.

Bruner, J. (1973). *Beyond the information given: Studies in the psychology of knowing.* New York: W. W. Norton.

Casper, L. (1990). Does family interaction prevent adolescent pregnancy? *Family Planning Perspectives, 22,* 109–114.

Chi, M., & Glaser, R. (1980). The measurement of expertise: Analysis of the development of knowledge and skills as a basis for assessing achievement. In E. L. Baker & E. S. Quellmatz (Eds.), *Educational testing and evaluation: Design, analyses, and policy* (pp. 37–47). Beverly Hills: Sage.

Condelli, L. (1986). Social and attitudinal determinants of contraceptive choice: Using the Health Belief Model. *The Journal of Sex Research, 22,* 478–491.

Cvetkovich, G., & Grote, B. (1983). Adolescent development and teenage fertility. In D. Byrne & W. Fisher (eds.), *Adolescents, sex, and contraception.* Hillsdale, NY: Lawrence Erlbaum Associates.

Danielson, R., Marcy, S., Plunkett, A., Wiest, W., & Greenlick, M. (1990). Reproductive health counseling for young men: What does it do? *Family Planning Perspectives, 22,* 115–121.

DiClemente, R., Durbin, M., Siegel, D., Krasnovsky, F., Lazarus, N., & Comacho, T. (1992). Determinants of condom use among junior high school students in a minority, inner-city school district. *Pediatrics, 89,* 197–202.

Eisen, M., Zellman, G., & McAlister, A. (1985). A health belief model approach to adolescents' fertility control: Some pilot program findings. *Health Education Quarterly, 12,* 185–210.

Eisen, M., Zellman, G., & McAlister, A. (1990). Evaluating the impact of a theory-based sexuality and contraceptive education program. *Family Planning Perspectives, 22*(6), 261–271.

Ewald, B., & Roberts, C. (1985). Contraceptive behavior in college-age males related to Fishbein model. *Advances in Nursing Science, 7*(3), 63–69.

Gibson, E. (1969). *Principles of perceptual learning and development.* New York: Appleton-Century-Crofts.

Goodman, E., & Cohall, A. (1989). Acquired immunodeficiency syndrome and adolescents: Knowledge, attitudes, beliefs, and behaviors in a New York City adolescent minority population. *Pediatrics, 84,* 36–42.

Graber, C. (1986). Contraceptive use in adolescent females and its relation to cognitive development status and identity formation. *Dissertation Abstracts International, 46,* 4400B. (University Microfilms No. AAD86–01778).

Green, V., Johnson, S., & Kaplan, D. (1992). Predictors of adolescent female decision making regarding contraceptive usage. *Adolescence, 27,* 613–631.

Hanna, K. (1990). Effect of nurse-client transaction on female adolescents' contraceptive perceptions and adherence. *Dissertations Abstracts International,* University of Pittsburgh.

Hanna, K. (1993). Effect of nurse-client transaction on female adolescents' oral contraceptive adherence. *IMAGE: Journal of Nursing Scholarship, 25,* 285–290.

Hanna, K. (1994). Female adolescents' perceived benefits and barriers to using oral contraceptives. *Issues in Comprehensive Pediatric Nursing, 17,* 47–55.

Hanna, K. (1995). Using King's theory of goal attainment to promote adolescents' health behavior. In M. Frey & C. Sieloff (Eds.), *Advancing King's conceptual framework and theory of goal attainment.* Newbury Park, CA: Sage.

Hayes-Roth, F., Klahr, P., & Mostoro, D. (1981). Advice taking and knowledge refinement: An iterative view of skill acquisition. In J. R. Anderson (Ed.), *Cognitive skills and their acquisition* (pp. 231–253). Hillsdale, NJ: Lawrence-Erlbaum.

Haynes, R. (1976). A critical review of the determinants of patient compliance with therapeutic regimens. In D. Sackett & R. Haynes (eds.), *Compliance with therapeutic regimens* (pp. 26–39). Baltimore: John Hopkins University Press.

Jaccard, J., & Becker, M. (1985). Attitude and behavior: An information integration perspective. *Journal of Experimental Social Psychology, 21,* 440–465.

Janz, N., & Becker, M. (1984). The Health Belief Model: A decade later. *Health Education Quarterly, 11,* 1–47.

Jemmott, L., & Jemmott, J. (1990). Sexual knowledge, attitudes, and risky sexual behavior among inner-city black male adolescents. *Journal of Adolescent Research, 5,* 346–369.

Joffe, A., & Radius, S. (1993). Self-efficacy and intent to use condoms among entering college freshman. *Journal of Adolescent Health, 14,* 262–268.

Kasch, C. (1986). Toward a theory of nursing action: Skills and competency in nurse-patient interaction. *Nursing Research, 35,* 226–230.

Kasch, C., & Knutson, K. (1985). Patient compliance and interpersonal style: Implications for practice and research. *Nurse Practitioner, 10,* 52–64.

Kasch, C., & Lisnek, P. (1984). The role of strategic communication in nursing theory and research. *Advances in Nursing Science, 7,* 56–71.

Kilman, P., Wanlass, R., Sabalis, R., & Sullivan, B. (1981). Sex education: A review of its effects. *Archives of Sexual Behavior, 10,* 177–205.

King, I. (1981). *A theory of nursing: Systems, concepts, process.* New York: Wiley.

Langley, P., & Simon, H. (1981). The central role of learning in cognition. In J. R. Anderson (Ed.), *Cognitive skills and their acquisition* (pp. 361–380). Hillsdale, NJ: Lawrence-Erlbaum.

Larkin, J., McDermott, J., Simon, D., & Simon, H. (1980). Expert and novice performance in solving physics problems. *Science, 208,* 1335–1342.

Leland, N., & Barth, R. (1992). Gender differences in knowledge, intentions, and behaviors concerning pregnancy and sexually transmitted disease prevention among adolescents. *Journal of Adolescent Health, 13,* 589–599.

Levine, M. (1971). *Renewal for nursing.* Philadelphia: F. A. Davis.

Levinson, R. A. (1995). Reproductive and contraceptive knowledge, contraceptive self-efficacy, and contraceptive behavior among teenage women. *Adolescence, 30*(11), 65–85.

Loewenstein, G., & Furstenberg, F. (1991). Is teenage sexual behavior rational? *Journal of Applied Social Psychology, 21,* 957–986.

Lowe, C., & Radius, S. (1987). Young adults' contraceptive practices: An investigation of influences. *Adolescence, 22,* 291–303.

Luker, K. (1975). *Taking chances: Abortion and the decision not to contracept.* Berkeley: University of California Press.

Marcy, S., Brown, J., & Danielson, R. (1983). Contraceptive use by adolescent females in relation to knowledge, and to time and method of contraceptive counseling. *Research in Nursing & Health, 6,* 175–182.

Martorano, S. (1977). A developmental analysis of performance on

Piaget's formal operations tasks. *Developmental Psychology, 13,* 666–672.

Maticka-Tyndale, E. (1991). Sexual scripts and AIDS prevention: Variations in adherence to safer-sex guidelines by heterosexual adolescents. *Journal of Sex Research, 28,* 45–66.

Mikhail, B. (1981). The health belief model: A review and critical evaluation of the model, research, and practice. *Advances in Nursing Science, 4,* 65–82.

Morrison, D. (1989). Predicting contraceptive efficacy: A discriminant analysis of three groups of adolescent women. *Journal of Applied Social Psychology, 19,* 1431–1452.

Namerow, P., Lawton, A., & Philliber, S. (1987). Teenagers' perceived and actual probabilities of pregnancy. *Adolescence, 22,* 475–485.

Namerow, P., Weatherby, N., & Williams-Kaye, J. (1989). The effectiveness of contingency-planning counseling. *Family Planning Perspectives, 21,* 115–119.

Nathanson, C., & Becker, M. (1985). The influence of client-provider relationships on teenage women's subsequent use of contraception. *American Journal of Public Health, 75,* 33–37.

Neimark, E. (1975). Intellectual development during adolescence. In. F. D. Horowitz (Ed.), *Review of child development research: Vol. 4* (pp. 541–594). Chicago: University of Chicago Press.

Neufeld, V. (1976). Patient education: A critique. In D. Sackett & R. Haynes (Eds.), *Compliance with Therapeutic Regimens* (pp. 83–92). Baltimore: John Hopkins University Press.

Newell, A., & Rosenbloom, P. (1981). Mechanisms of skill acquisition and the law of practice. In J. R. Anderson (Ed.), *Cognitive skills and their acquisition* (pp. 1–56). Hillsdale, NJ: Lawrence-Erlbaum.

Nisbett, R., & Ross, L. (1980). *Human inference: Strategies and shortcomings of social judgment.* Englewood Cliffs, NJ: Prentice-Hall.

Norris, A. (1988). Cognitive analysis of contraceptive behavior. *IMAGE: Journal of Nursing Scholarship, 20,* 135–140.

Orlando, I. (1972). *The discipline and teaching of nursing process.* New York: G. P. Putnam's Sons.

Orr, D., & Langefeld, C. (1993). Factors associated with condom use by sexually active male adolescents at risk for sexually transmitted disease. *Pediatrics, 91,* 873–879.

Paterson J., & Zderad, L. (1976). *Humanistic nursing.* New York: Wiley.

Peplau, H. (1952). *Interpersonal relations in nursing: A conceptual frame of reference for psychodynamic nursing.* New York: G. P. Putman's Sons.

Pleck, J., Sonenstein, F., & Ku, L. (1990). Contraceptive attitudes and intention to use condoms in sexually experienced and inexperienced adolescent males. *Journal of Family Issues, 11,* 294–312.

Piaget, J. (1972). Intellectual evolution from adolescence to adulthood. *Human Development, 15,* 1–12.

Redeker, N. (1988). Health beliefs and adherence in chronic illness. *IMAGE: Journal of Nursing Scholarship, 20,* 31–35.

Rodin, J., & Janis, I. (1979). The social power of health-care practitioners as agents of change. *Journal of Social Issues, 35,* 60–81.

Rosenstock, I. (1966). Why people use health sources. *Milbank Memorial Quarterly, 44,* 94–124.

Rubin, R. (1968). A theory of clinical nursing. *Nursing Research, 17,* 210–212.

Sachs, B. (1985). Contraceptive decision–making in urban, black female adolescents: Its relationship to cognitive development. *International Journal of Nursing, 22,* 117–126.

Smith, P., Beck, J., & Davies, D. (1987). Contraceptive use among high-risk adolescents. *Journal of Sex Education and Therapy, 13,* 52–57.

Strader, M., & Beaman, M. (1989). College students' knowledge about AIDS and attitudes toward condom use. *Public Health Nursing, 6,* 62–66.

Tanfer, K., Grady, W., Klepinger, D., & Billy, J. (1993). Condom use among U.S. men, 1991. *Family Planning Perspectives, 25,* 61–66.

Tanfer, K., & Rosenbaum, E. (1986). Contraceptive perceptions and method choice among young single women in the United States. *Studies in Family Planning, 17,* 269–277.

Tomlinson-Keasey, C. (1972). Formal operations in females from eleven to fifty-four years of age. *Developmental Psychology, 6,* 364.

Voss, J. (1980). Sex education: Evaluation and recommendations for future study. *Archives of Sexual Behavior, 9,* 37–59.

Weisman, C., Plichta, S., Nathanson, C., Chase, G., Ensminger, M., & Robinson, J. (1991). Adolescent women's contraceptive decision making. *Journal of Health and Social Behavior, 32,* 130–144.

White, J. (1984). Initiating contraceptive use: How do young women decide? *Pediatric Nursing, 10,* 347–352.

Whitley, B., & Schofield, J. (1985, 1986). A meta-analysis of research on adolescent contraceptive use. *Population and Environment, 8,* 173–203.

Zabin, L., Stark, H., & Emerson, M. (1991). Reasons for delay in contraceptive clinic utilization. *Journal of Adolescent Health, 12,* 225–232.

Characteristics of Specific Populations and Contraceptive Use

The chapters in this part focus on characteristics of contraceptive users that are influential to their effective use of and their experience with using contraceptives. Chapter 4 describes aspects of culture and class that influence the methods women and men will choose and feel comfortable using. Many factors related to contraceptive methods are in opposition to strongly felt cultural beliefs. Class is an important factor in determining access to knowledge, contraceptive methods, and the health care system. Chapter 5 describes the limited knowledge that is available on men who are contraceptive users. Men's direct involvement in contraception is limited due to the few methods within their direct control. However, men are influential in their partners' contraceptive use. Chapter 6 focuses on adolescents as novice contraceptors because of their limited experience with contraception and their level of development. Chapter 7 deals with midlife women who have not become infertile through sterilization or hysterectomy, and how they work with their waning level of fertility. As women age and experience physiological changes, various methods become contraindicated. It is also difficult to know the times when women may be fertile and when they are anovulatory.

The Influence of Culture and Socioeconomic Status on Contraceptive Use

Dona J. Lethbridge

Culture, and associated factors such as ethnicity, race, and socio-economic status (SES) or class have inestimable influence on contraceptive choices, use, and access. This chapter will focus on the influences of differences from the mainstream American culture—how specific cultural groups might differ in their contraceptive choice and use, as well as childbearing norms, and how they might be viewed and treated by the health care system.

MAINSTREAM AMERICAN CULTURE AND FERTILITY REGULATION

American culture is suffused with messages and expectations about the value of sexual behavior that is unplanned, romantic, and frequent. Sexuality is used in advertisements to sell merchandise, portrayed frankly on television and in the movies, and revealed in women's fashions. Yet, at the same time, teenagers are expected to abstain from sexual activity (though premarital sexual behavior in adults is unspokenly acceptable); and, though contraception cannot, with good manners, be mentioned in public, pregnancies should occur only when planned and within marriage. Abortion is legally obtainable through the second trimester, but considered completely unacceptable by a large segment of society, and generally distasteful by those who believe in the right to its availability (Luker, 1984).

The most frequently used contraceptive method in the United States by women aged 15 to 44 is sterilization, either their own or their partners'. A close second is hormonal contraception, whether birth control pills, progestin (e.g., Depo Provera) injections, or progestin (e.g., Norplant) implants. Both of these methods are disassociated from sexual behavior.

Preferences and perceptions are substantially formed through cultural and familial socialization. However, accessibility to services and availability of contraceptive methods also determine how effective women and their partners may be in preventing unwanted pregnancy. This chapter presents a list of attributes of American culture (see Table 4.1). They may be assumed to be normal for those living in this country, yet may, in fact, be far different for those having been socialized in the ways of other cultures. Some attributes will influence the kinds of contraception considered acceptable, some how diligently it will be used to prevent pregnancy, and some how women and men might relate to and be perceived by professionals within the health care system.

CULTURAL FACTORS INFLUENCING CONTRACEPTIVE CHOICE AND USE

A number of cultural norms and beliefs will influence which contraceptives will be tolerable to women and men, and how they will feel and be treated as they deal with the health care system. Women's feelings about their body, and especially a reluctance to touch their genitalia, will make barrier methods such as foam or the diaphragm unusable. This is an important factor for Asian women. In Taiwan, a rapidly developing country with a very active government-sponsored family planning program, the diaphragm is not available as a contraceptive choice (Lethbridge, 1995; Lethbridge & Wang, 1992).* Indeed, women in that relatively modern country do not use tampons during menses. Kulig (1988) describes Cambodian women's birth control use and notes their aversion to methods such as the IUD, the diaphragm, and foam since they require women to touch themselves.

---

*From Lethbridge, D. J. (1995). Fertility management in Taiwanese and African-American women. *Journal of Obstetrical, Gynecologic and Neonatal Nursing, 24,* 459–463. Copyright © 1995 by Lippincott-Raven. Adapted with permission.

TABLE 4.1. Cultural Contrasts Between Mainstream American Culture and Some Other World Cultures that Might Influence Contraceptive Use[a]

Control versus fatalism
U.S. Culture: Individuals have the power to control the future.
Other Cultures: The future is influenced by fate or by a higher power.
Seven-eighths of the world's population believes in fatalism.

Control of nature versus harmony with nature
U.S. Culture: Nature can, and should be, controlled and used to meet human needs.
Other Cultures: Humans are part of nature and should disturb it as little as possible.

Change versus tradition
U.S. Culture: Change is usually good.
Other Cultures: Change should be resisted unless there is an obvious good to be gained from abandoning tradition.

The importance of the future versus the past and present
U.S. Culture: It is important to plan for and anticipate the future.
Other Cultures: It is important to remember the past and enjoy the present moment.

Reality is orderly versus reality is disorderly
U.S. Culture: All reality can eventually be categorized and ordered.
Other Cultures: Reality is chaos and cannot be objectively organized.

Guilt versus shame
U.S. Culture: Acts are to be avoided out of fear of internal feelings of guilt.
Other Cultures: Acts are to be avoided out of fear of public shame.

Practicality versus aesthetics and emotions
U.S. Culture: Practicality and pragmatic ends are more important than emotions or aesthetic considerations.
Other Cultures: Aesthetics and emotions are at least of equal value to practicality.

Rational versus intuitive thinking
U.S. Culture: The most productive thinking is linear, cause and effect, and rational in nature; it is based on concrete evidence and facts.
Other Cultures: Intuitive, creative thinking is most highly valued.

Becoming versus being
U.S. Culture: People should constantly strive to become better.
Other Cultures: There is value in simply existing as one is, rather than constantly striving to become something else.

Speed and time as priority versus time as secondary
U.S. Culture: Efficiency, scheduling, punctuality, and speed are of paramount importance.

(cont.)

TABLE 4.1. *(Continued)*

Other Cultures: Units of time are undifferentiated and are only rarely an important consideration.

Independence versus dependence
U.S. Culture: It is unhealthy to be dependent on family and the group.
Other Cultures: It is proper to remain dependent on the family and group into and throughout adulthood.

Questioning versus respecting authority
U.S. Culture: It is all right, even desirable, to question authority figures.
Other Cultures: It is wrong to question any authority figures.

Achievements versus character
U.S. Culture: Individuals are valued according to their external achievements.
Other Cultures: Individuals are to be judged not according to their external achievements, but by their general character and inner self.

Complaints versus reluctance to complain
U.S. Culture: It is all right, and desirable, to a point, to complain to one's superiors.
Other Cultures: It is defiant of authority to complain to superiors.

Direct versus indirect questioning
U.S. Culture: Direct questioning is the best way to get information.
Other Cultures: Direct questioning is rude and intrusive.

Direct answers versus softened responses
U.S. Culture: Direct answers, even if they are negative, are efficient and tend to be respected.
Other Cultures: Direct negative responses should be avoided because they cause loss of face and disharmony and are rude.

Informality versus formality
U.S. Culture: Informality and casual appearance are signs of warmth and equality.
Other Cultures: Informality can be intrusive and can result in loss of respect for a superior.

Variety versus consistency of procedures
U.S. Culture: Constant efforts should be made to find new and better ways to do tasks.
Other Cultures: Once a procedure has been worked out, it should not be changed unless absolutely necessary.

[a] Adapted from: Thiederman, S. (1991).

Menstrual beliefs are also important in their influence on the use of hormonal contraceptives. The birth control pill and injectable contraceptives often lighten menstrual flow, and hormonal implants often cause menses to decrease altogether after about a year of use. Many cultures view menses as the body ridding itself of toxins or "bad blood." A light or absent flow means that the toxins stay in the body or, in the words of Cambodian women, become "stuck blood," a condition to be avoided at all costs (Kulig, 1988). The IUD, on the other hand, may increase menstrual flow, but this would not be viewed as a problem. Women in Taiwan and the Peoples' Republic of China use the IUD predominantly as their contraceptive method (Kaufman, Zhang, Qiao, & Ahang, 1992; Lethbridge & Wang, 1992).

Marital and childbearing patterns will influence when contraception will be adopted. Some cultures, such as the United States, tolerate premarital intercourse, and expect sexually active couples, even adolescents, to use an effective contraceptive method. Cultures in Africa also tolerate premarital intercourse, but are comfortable if a pregnancy should ensue and do not expect contraceptive use. It is not unusual, however, for cultures to postpone sexual activity, to marry late, to have children as they arrive after the marriage, and then to begin contraceptive use after their family is considered complete. In western countries, the pattern is to delay pregnancy after marriage, and to optimally space children thereafter. Therefore, there is an emphasis on the importance of "planning" pregnancy in mainstream western culture, a desire that is irrelevant to many other cultures. These varying childbearing patterns influence contraceptive use in that sterilization may be more readily used after the family is considered complete, or abortions may be used during a woman's later years rather than during the childbearing years to space pregnancy (Lethbridge & Wang, 1992).

Male and female roles in decision making regarding contraceptive choice and childbearing are also relevant. In the United States, the trend is for women to take responsibility for contraception, since they are the ones who are concerned about the burden of conceiving an unwanted pregnancy (Lethbridge, 1991). Relationships in the United States might well be relatively egalitarian, in that women, occupationally active and financially independent, will have equal say in decisions in the relationship. In other countries, women might be financially dependent on their husbands, as well as expected to obey his wishes. In some cultures, a large number of children are still considered necessary for family work and to guarantee care of aging parents. More sons are especially valued (Callon & Kee, 1981). A man may see childbearing as a sign of virility, leading him to discourage his wife's use of contraception and to resist the use of vasectomy. This perspective of child-bearing may be present in subcultures of the United States, in, for instance, the case of young African American men (Rivara, Sweeney, & Henderson, 1985).

Myths and beliefs about conception will also influence contraceptive choice. Asian women consider that a body must be "cool" to conceive a pregnancy (Kulig, 1988). If the man's body is also "cool," pregnancy is even more likely. A state of coolness could be attained by eating such foods as green vegetables, bean curd, and cold noodles. Amenorrhea would lead to a condition that is "hot." Some Cambodian women reported that the birth control pill made them dizzy and "hot" (Kulig, 1988).

The belief in fatalism will influence the diligence with which contraception is adopted and used. If the number and arrival of one's children are preordained, as for example in the Hispanic culture, fewer attempts will be made to change events (Marin et al., 1993; Grady, Klepinger, & Billy, 1993). Those believing in Hindi doctrine also may believe that they are predestined to have a specific number of children. Events in past lives might lead to the reward of bearing many children in a current life (Kurian & Ghosh, 1983).

Specific potions might be used to prevent pregnancy, such as certain shrubs or roots (sometimes purgatives) to chew or in tea taken after sexual intercourse by Botswanans (Schapera, 1978). In Cambodian culture, a burning ceremony is performed by a healer, where incense is used to burn specific areas of the abdomen in women, where it is thought to seal the fallopian tubes, and in men (Kulig, 1988).

Religious norms and restrictions may be considered cultural prohibitions regarding birth control and as prevalent for mainstream Americans as those of other cultures. Roman Catholics, for example, are prohibited from sexual behavior that may not result in a conception, and thus all birth control is prohibited except abstinence during fertile days. Thus, natural family planning may be used by devout Roman Catholics. This prohibition, however, may still be perceived to permit women and men to use birth control methods that result in "minimal sin" such as undergoing sterilization, a one-time experience, or having an IUD inserted. Those of the Mormon faith believe the more children you have the closer to God you get. They would thus be reluctant to limit their family size (Conley, 1990). On the other hand, those individuals of faiths prohibiting abortion, such as Roman Catholic and Fundamentalist Protestant, even when living in poverty, have been found to have lower levels of unwanted pregnancies (see Table 4.2).

Varying socioeconomic classes may also be considered cultural groups. It is clear that those living in poverty have increased numbers of

TABLE 4.2.   Contraceptive Failures During the First 12 Months of Use,
Reported by Race/Ethnicity, Religion, and Poverty Status

Race, ethnicity, and religion	Total (%)	< 200% of poverty level	> 200% of poverty level
Total	13.78	21.2	10.3
Race and Ethnicity			
White	12.7	22.4	12.5
African American	17.6	30.8	17.6
Hispanic	16.4	28.7	16.3
Religion			
Catholic	13.4	20.6	9.9
Fundamentalist Protestant	11.4	15.2	9.6
Other	15.4	24.8	10.8

Source: Adapted with the permission of The Alan Guttmacher Institute from William D. Mosher. "Contraceptive Practice in the United States, 1982–1988." *Family Planning Perspectives.* Volume 22, Number 5. September/October 1990.

unwanted pregnancies, with a concomitant lack of access to contraception (see Table 4.2). The National Survey of Family Growth (N.S.F.G.), in 1988, described 10.3% of births within the previous five years were described as unwanted at the time of conception by the mother (Williams & Pratt, 1990). The percentage of unwanted conceptions for African American women was higher than the general population of women, at 22.8%. Further, the proportion of unwanted births rose between 1982 and 1988, from 7.7 to 10.3% This is most pronounced among women living in poverty, where the proportion of unwanted births rose by almost 75%, from 10.2 to 17.4%. In 1988, the percentage of unwanted pregnancies among poor African American women was more than double that of poor white women, at 35% for African American and 17% for white women. It could be speculated that as the United States has gone through a recession in the 1980s, financial hardship has been exacerbated for the poor.

Simmons and Elias (1994) describe issues related to family planning client and provider interactions and note the status differential between many women and men and the professionals who treat them. This is especially apparent when clients are poor, and exaggerated when they are people of color. Therefore, not only will decreased income make contraception inaccessible, but less than optimal treatment by clinics may make women and men reluctant to attend them, and they may have less access to sources of contraceptive knowledge such as schooling and access to the media. Literacy may also be an issue with the very poor. In very low-income, rural areas of the southeastern United States, the mean literacy level has been found to be third grade (Jackson et al., 1991). Literacy levels of standard contraceptive pamphlets and brochures have been found to be at tenth to twelfth grade (Swanson et al., 1990; Williams-Deane & Potter, 1992). Finally, many cultural attributes among those listed in Table 4.1 will influence interactions with health care professionals. Native Americans, for example, a set of subcultural groups within the United States, share attributes that relate to respect for authority figures and a reluctance to question them, a more harmonious relationship with their world and events that befall them, and a different perspective on time and the present. Native American adolescents have been found to be more sexually active, to have more adolescent births, and to be half as likely to use contraception than their non-native peers (Digest, 1992a). The effects of poverty and cultural characteristics, such that they are unable to deal effectively with the health care system, might contribute to these differences.

Upper socioeconomic class may also influence contraceptive choice and use. In a study of professional, affluent women, it was found that they had fewer unwanted pregnancies than American women generally, and tended to use less theoretically effective methods and to use them successfully (Lethbridge, 1990). It can be speculated that there is less status differential between these women and men and health care professionals, and thus they are able to use the health care system very well to meet their needs. Similarly, in studies of women in other countries, those women with educational and occupational success have lower fertility rates, in spite of less effective contraception such as barrier methods, rhythm, and withdrawal (see Table 4.3). Kasarda, Billy, and West (1986) have reviewed the literature on fertility and SES, and found that fertility levels have decreased as affluence and literacy levels increase.

THE EXPERIENCE OF AFRICAN AMERICAN WOMEN

Because African Americans are such an important and substantive part of the American population, they may be used as an example of a cultural group somewhat different from, but inextricably a part of mainstream American culture. Many, if not most, African Americans are from families that have lived in the United States for six genera-

TABLE 4.3.   Contraceptive Methods of Women in European Countries
with Low Fertility Rates, 1984–1985 (%)

Method	Italy	Spain	France	West Germany	Great Britain
IUD	15	13	18	1	7
Pill/injectables	6	19	32	34	37
Sterilization					
Both sexes	0	3	5	8	25
Barrier methods	23	23	9	8	17
Withdrawal	14	9	6	1	3
Rhythm	12	6	6	13	1
No method	30	26	24	19	10

Source: Adapted with permission of The Alan Guttmacher Institute from Margarita Delgado Pérez and Massimo Livi-Bacci. "Fertility in Italy and Spain: The Lowest in the World." *Family Planning Perspectives.* Volume 24, Number 4, July/August 1992.

tions or more. Moreover, they are expected to conform to the values and norms of the dominant culture, and, in fact, arguments have been made as to whether there is a distinct culture unique to African Americans (Hill, 1972). In studies comparing the two cultures, however, differences can be identified. In describing African American culture, Butts (1981), an African American sex educator, described it as having a more "sex-positive" view of life than mainstream culture. She included a description of African American families as more sensuous, that is, interpreting the world through the senses: sight, sound, taste, smell, and touch. Children grow up with physical affection and adults touch each other in friendship. In addition, given the history of many African Americans, from forbears that lived in slavery, the importance of kinship and family remains a formidable force. Survival has meant taking care of each other and staying close within the community. Since blood ties historically were often unclear, family may include friends or a new community may become a family. Similarly, fecundity is valued. "A baby is the future," and one proves one's worth through childbearing. Abortion is used less by African American women than women generally in the United States (Henshaw, Koonin, & Smith, 1991) and legal, anonymous adoption is rare (Bachrach, Stolley, & London, 1992).

Women are dominant in African American families, raising their own children, and at times, their grandchildren and the children of friends and other family. African American women begin sexual activity and childbearing earlier than mainstream U.S. women, and are less likely to be married when bearing children. There are fewer African American men available for marriage, through inclination, incarceration, as well as higher mortality rate for younger men, so more families are headed by women alone. Given the dearth of men, it is understandable that childbearing without marriage would be an acceptable and practical alternative.

It is important, however, to include the effect of poverty and socioeconomic status when describing behavior. While African American teenage births are considered to be at high risk for low birth rate, underweight births have been found to be equally likely among both African American and white women living below the U.S. poverty level (Digest, 1992b). Edelman and Pittman (1986) write that young African American women and men have less access to contraceptive information and services, and see no compelling reasons to delay parenthood. Young African American men are more likely to father children when teenage pregnancies are frequent in their community, accepted, and when they perceive fatherhood to be minimally disruptive to their lives (Rivara, Sweeney, & Henderson, 1985). When educational experiences seem unsuccessful and occupational opportunities few, parenthood would be an avenue for reward, admiration, and self-worth. It is noteworthy that in early research by Zelnik, Kantner, and Ford (1981) of American teenagers' sexual behavior and contraceptive use, among the most effective contraceptors were middle-class African American girls. It could be speculated that their families, successful within the dominant culture, not only imparted mainstream cultural values to their daughters, but saw for them educational and occupational successes that would be hindered by childbearing.

African American women have differing patterns of contraceptive use than mainstream women (Mosher, 1990) (see Table 4.2). Tubal sterilization is by far the dominant contraceptive method for this group, with male sterilization rare. Equal numbers of women use hormonal contraception. Less dominant are barrier methods. There has been little study of contraceptive choices of African American women and the predominant use of female sterilization is notable. Questions may be raised as to the extent of informed consent some African American women may have made; that is, were they covertly coerced because of their marital and childbearing status? A greater use of sterilization, however, may also reflect their partners' reluctance to undergo vasectomy, more predominant among mainstream U.S. men. It may also be a result of earlier childbearing and an earlier attainment of desired family size, so that sterilization is a practical solution.

STRATEGIES FOR INTERVENTION

Health care providers need to keep an open mind when counseling women and couples on contraception. A purported similarity to an American lifestyle does not guarantee that behavior will conform to mainstream American values. With the many migrant and immigrant groups moving into the United States, providers are ever more likely to be working with other cultural groups, with differing childbearing and contraceptive norms and expectations. Nor should a pattern of child-bearing that differs from the mainstream be automatically assumed to be unsatisfactory. It may be consistent with the context within which the woman lives and most comfortable, in spite of inconsistencies with mainstream expectations.

REFERENCES

Bachrach, C. A., Stolley, K. S., & London, K. A. (1992). Relinquishment of premarital births: Evidence from national survey data. *Family Planning Perspectives, 24,* 27–32.

Butts, J. D. (1981). Adolescent sexuality and teenage pregnancy from a Black perspective. In T. Ooms, (ed.) *Teenage pregnancy in a family context* (pp. 307–325). Philadelphia: Temple University Press.

Callon, V. J., & Kee, P. (1981). Sons or daughters? Cross-cultural comparisons of the sex preferences of Australian, Greek, Italian Malay, Chinese and Indian parents in Australia and Malaysia. *Population and Environment, 4*(2), 97–102.

Conley, L. J. (1990). Childbearing and childrearing practices in Mormonism. *Neonatal Network, 9*(3), 41–48.

Digest. (1992a). Among Native American teenagers, sex without contraceptives is common. *Family Planning Perspectives, 24,* 189–191.

Digest. (1992b). Underweight births are equally likely among poor blacks and whites. *Family Planning Perspectives, 24,* 95–96.

Edelman, M. W., & Pittman, K. J. (1986). Adolescent pregnancy: Black and white. *Journal of Community Health, 11,* 63–69.

Grady, W. R., Klepinger, D. H., & Billy, J. O. (1993). The influence of community characteristics on the practice of effective contraception. *Family Planning Perspectives, 25*(1), 4–11.

Henshaw, S. K., Koonin, L. M., & Smith, J. C. (1991). Characteristics of U.S. women having abortions, 1987. *Family Planning Perspectives, 23*(2), 75–81.

Henshaw, S. K., Koonin, L. M., & Van Vort, J. (1987). Characteristics of

U.S. women having abortions, 1987. *Family Planning Perspectives, 23*, 75–78.

Hill, R. (1972). *The strength of black families.* New York: Emerson Hall Press.

Jackson, R. H., Davis, T. C., Bairnsfather, L. E., George, R. B., Crouch, M. A., & Gault, H. (1991). Patient reading ability: An overlooked problem in health care. *Southern Medical Journal, 84*, 1172–1175.

Jones, E. F., & Forrest, J. D. (1992). Contraceptive failure rates based on the 1988 N.S.F.G. *Family Planning Perspectives, 24*, 1219.

Kasarda, J. D., Billy, J. O. D., & West, K. (1986). *Status enhancement and fertility.* New York: Academic.

Kaufman, J., Zhang, Z., Qiao, X., & Zhang, Y. (1992). The quality of family planning services in rural China. *Studies in Family Planning, 23*(2), 73–84.

Kulig, J. C. (1988). Conception and birth control use: Cambodian refugee women's beliefs and practices. *Journal of Community Health Nursing, 5*, 235–246.

Kurian, G., & Ghosh, R. (1983). Child-rearing in transition in Indian immigration families in Canada. *Journal of Comparative Family Studies, 83*, 132–133.

Lethbridge, D. J. (1990). Use of contraceptives by women of upper socioeconomic status. *Health Care for Women International, 11*, 305–318.

Lethbridge, D. J. (1991). Choosing and using contraception: Toward a theory of women's contraceptive self-care. *Nursing Research, 40*, 276–280.

Lethbridge, D. J. (1995). Fertility management in Taiwanese and African-American women. *Journal of Obstetrical, Gynecologic and Neonatal Nursing, 24*, 459–463.

Lethbridge, D. J., & Wang, R. (1992). Patterns of contraceptive use of women in Taiwan. *Health Care for Women International, 12*, 431–441.

Luker, K. (1984). *Abortion and the politics of motherhood.* Berkeley, CA: University of California Press.

Mosher, W. D. (1990). Contraceptive practice in the United States, 1982–1988. *Family Planning Perspectives, 22*, 198–205.

Perez, M. D., & Livi-Bacci, M. (1992). Fertility in Italy and Spain: The lowest in the world. *Family Planning Perspectives, 24*, 162–171.

Rivara, F. P., Sweeney, P. J., & Henderson, B. F. (1985). A study of low socioeconomic status, Black teenage fathers and their nonfather peers. *Pediatrics, 75*, 648–656.

Schapera, I. (1978). Some Kgatla theories of procreation. In J. Argyle & E. Preston-Whyte (Eds.), *Social systems and traditions in South Africa.* Capetown: Oxford University Press.

Simmons, R., & Elias, C. (1994). The study of client-provider interactions: A review of methodological issues. *Studies in Family Planning, 25,* 1–17.

Swanson, J., Forrest, K., Ledbetter, C., Hall, S., Holstine, E., & Shafer, M. (1990). Readability of commercial and generic contraceptive instructions. *Image: Journal of Nursing Scholarship, 22,* 96–100.

Thiederman, S. (1991). *Bridging cultural barriers for corporate success.* New York: Lexington Press.

Williams, L. B., & Pratt, W. F. (1990). Wanted and unwanted childbearing in the United States: 1973–1988. *Advance data from vital and health statistics of the national center for health statistics, no. 189.* Hyattsville, MD: National Center for Health Statistics.

Williams-Deane, M., & Potter, L. (1992). Current oral contraceptive use instructions: An analysis of patient package inserts. *Family Planning Perspectives, 24,* 111–115.

Zelnik, M., Kantner, J. F., & Ford K. (1981). *Sex and pregnancy in adolescence.* Beverly Hills, CA: Sage Publications.

CHAPTER FIVE

Males: Partners in Contraception

Kathleen M. Hanna

This chapter discusses the limited knowledge on males and contraception. Contraceptive use is usually reported for females from which male use is inferred. This is probably related to society's recognition that males are partners in conception, but not in contraception (Lethbridge, 1991; Swanson, 1985). If male contraceptive use has been studied, the population was usually adolescents and the method was condoms. However, males are directly involved in several contraceptive methods (condom, vasectomy, withdrawal, and abstinence) and indirectly involved (as influential partners) in others (Gallen, Liskin, & Kak, 1986). Males have an influence on their partners' contraceptive use (Zotti & Siegel, 1995).

There is some knowledge of male sexual behavior. However, it is not the intent of this chapter to review antecedents to sexual behavior. For reviews of male sexual behavior, the reader is referred to Marsiglio (1988).

SEXUAL BEHAVIOR

Sexual behavior becomes significant with the possibility of reproduction. At puberty, childhood levels of testosterone increase and no longer inhibit the hypothalamus thus producing gonadotropins. In turn, testosterone production is stimulated (Tanner, 1971). The higher testosterone levels stimulate secondary sex characteristic development and reproductive organ maturation. Changes include growth of testes,

65

TABLE 5.1. Percentage of Unmarried Male
Adolescents in the United States Who Have
Had Sexual Intercourse at Least Once

	Year	
Years of age	1979	1988
15		33
16		50
17		66
18		72
19		86
15–19		60
17–19	66	76

Source: Reproduced with permission of The Alan Guttmacher
Institute from Freyal L. Sonenstein, Joseph H. Pleck and Leighton
C. Ku. "Sexual Activity, Condom Use and AIDS Awareness Among
Adolescent Males." *Family Planning Perspectives,* Vol. 21, No. 4.
July/August 1989.

scrotum, and penis; appearance of axillary, facial, and pubic hair; and
temporary development of breast tissue (for some).

ADOLESCENT SEXUAL ACTIVITY

The majority initiate sexual intercourse during adolescence and the
portion has increased between 1979 and 1988 (see Table 5.1). Initiation
of sexual intercourse increases with age. African Americans have first
sexual intercourse at earlier ages than whites (nonHispanic) and Hispanics (Ku, Sonenstein, & Pleck, 1993), with the average age being 11 to
12 years (Clark, Zabin, & Hardy, 1984; Jemmott & Jemmott, 1990).

Several behaviors typify adolescents' sexual relationships. Serial
monogamy, a sexual relationship with only one person for an uncertain
length of time, is common (Netting, 1992; Sorenson, 1973). The majority
(79%) are involved in only one sexual relationship at a time (Sonenstein, Pleck, & Ku, 1991). However, they have an average of five sexual
partners in their adolescent lifetime (Sonenstein et al., 1991). Sexual
intercourse is infrequent, with the average 15- to 19-year-old male having sexual intercourse 2.7 times a month (Sonenstein et al., 1991).

ADULT SEXUAL ACTIVITY

The majority have had vaginal intercourse (see Table 5.2). These men
have had a median of 4.7 vaginal sexual encounters in the past 4 weeks

TABLE 5.2. **Percentage of 20- to 30-Year-Old Males
in the United States Who Have Had Sexual
Intercourse at Least Once**

Type of sex	1991 (%)
Vaginal intercourse	95
Anal intercourse	20
Performed oral sex	75
Received oral sex	79

Source: Reproduced with permission of The Alan Guttmacher Institute from John O. G. Billy, Koray Tanfer, William R. Grady and Daniel H. Klepinger. "The Sexual Behavior of Men in the United States." *Family Planning Perspectives.* Vol. 25, No. 2. March/April 1993.

and 7.3 vaginal sexual partners in their lifetime (Billy et al., 1993). The number of vaginal sexual partners increases with age (Billy et al., 1993).

CONTRACEPTIVE BEHAVIOR

ADOLESCENTS AND CONTRACEPTION

The predominant contraceptive method is condoms, with the majority using them alone or with other methods (see Table 5.3). Other methods may be withdrawal and oral contraceptives (OCs). Withdrawal was used by 10% and 7% and OCs was used by 9% and 27% at first and last sexual intercourse respectively (Pleck, Sonenstein, & Swain, 1988).

Contraceptive use varies with age and progresses toward more effective methods. Condom use is greater for those who initiate intercourse at an older age (see Table 5.4). However, with age, condom use

TABLE 5.3. **Percentage of 17- to 19-Year-Old Males Using
Contraceptive Methods at Last Sexual Intercourse**

Contraceptive method	1979 (%)	1988 (%)
Condom alone or with other contraception	21	58
Effective female contraception without condom	28	22
Ineffective or no contraception	51	21

Source: Reproduced with permission of The Alan Guttmacher Institute from Freyal L. Sonenstein, Joseph H. Pleck and Leighton C. Ku. "Sexual Activity, Condom Use and AIDS Awareness Among Adolescent Males." *Family Planning Perspectives.* Vol. 21. No. 4. July/August 1989.

TABLE 5.4.   Percentage of 15- to 19-Year-Old Males Using
Contraceptive Methods at First Sexual Intercourse

Contraceptive method	Age			
	< 12	12–14	15–17	18–19
Condom alone or with other contraception	17	48	61	64
Effective female contraception without condom	9	3	8	20
Ineffective or no contraception	74	48	32	16

Source: Reproduced with the permission of The Alan Guttmacher Institute from Freyal L. Sonenstein, Joseph H. Pleck and Leighton C. Ku. "Sexual Activity, Condom Use and AIDS Awareness Among Adolescent Males." *Family Planning Perspectives.* Vol. 21, No. 4. July/August 1989.

decreases (Pleck, Sonenstein, & Ku, 1993). Being older is associated with greater condom use at first sexual intercourse and lower condom use at last sexual intercourse (Pleck et al., 1988). Those who used a condom at first sexual intercourse changed to a female method, and those who did not use contraception at first intercourse changed to condoms at last intercourse (Pleck et al., 1988).

Condom use may be seen predominantly as a means to prevent pregnancy. Condom use is negatively associated with OCs (Maticka-Tyndale, 1991; Pleck et al., 1991). However, the AIDS epidemic may be influencing condom use. Condom use has increased considerably between 1979 and 1988 (see Table 5.4). Further, consistent condom use and use with last partner has increased between 1988 and 1991 (Pleck et al., 1993).

Contraceptive use is associated with sociodemographic and situational factors. Contraceptive use is less for those who did not use it at first intercourse, were going steady or engaged to their partner, and were African American (Pleck et al., 1988), and is greater for those who have frequent sexual intercourse (Gold & Berger, 1983). Condom use is less with those who are young and have had three partners in the past year (Pleck et al., 1991); however, condom use is greater for African Americans (Pleck et al., 1988, 1991). Use of female contraceptive methods is associated with higher actual or aspired education (Pleck et al., 1988).

ADULTS AND CONTRACEPTION

A minority of adults use condoms. This may be influenced by marital status and commitment. Fewer married (18%) than single men (39%)

use condoms. Further, condom use decreases as commitment in a relationship increases. For example, condom use is less likely among married than unmarried men; cohabiting than single men with a regular partner; and single men with a regular partner than without one (Tanfer et al., 1993). In addition, condom use is greater among men with multiple partners and in a one-night stand (Tanfer et al., 1993). In men, condom use also decreases with age. Of those aged 20 to 24, usage is 39%; 25 to 29, it is 33%; 30 to 34, 21%; and 35 to 39, 17% (Tanfer et al., 1993).

Condom use varies with how it is measured, by sexual behavior, and sexual partners. Always using condoms is as low as 9% (Catania et al., 1992). Condom use is greater for bisexuals and homosexuals than for heterosexuals (Tanfer et al., 1993), and for adults than adolescents (Anderson, Freese, & Pennbridge, 1994). Always using condoms is lower (29%) with vaginal sex than with anal sex (50%) (Thomas & Hodges, 1991). Condom use is greater with a secondary rather than with a primary partner among males with multiple partners (Marin, Gomez, & Hearst, 1993). For STD clients, condom use is greater for males with casual partners than with primary or regular partners (Centers for Disease Control [CDC], 1993).

RISK-TAKING BEHAVIOR

Contraceptive and sexual behavior is related to risk-taking behavior. High-risk sexual behavior, which includes lack of condom use, is associated with alcohol and drug use among adolescents (Biglan et al., 1990; Hingson et al., 1990; Jemmott & Jemmott, 1993; Keller et al., 1991; Orr & Langefeld, 1993). In one study, greater than half of adolescents had sexual intercourse when using alcohol or drugs, with about half of them not using contraception (Leland & Barth, 1992).

MASCULINITY AND CONTRACEPTION

Males hold various beliefs about male roles and contraceptive responsibility. Adolescents believe in male responsibility (Marsiglio, 1993; Pleck et al., 1990, 1991) and in both male and female responsibility (Pleck et al., 1988). Only a minority (10%) believe that they would be pleased if they impregnated a partner (Marsiglio, 1993). In addition, only a minority (21%) believe that impregnating a partner would make them "feel like a real man" (Marsiglio, 1993), and this belief declined between 1988 and 1991 (Pleck et al., 1993). Beliefs about male roles and responsibility may be interrelated. For example, belief that impregnating their partner would make them "feel like a real man" is greater among those who held more traditional beliefs about male roles (Marsiglio, 1993).

Male contraceptive use has been associated with beliefs about masculinity and male roles. Males who believe in male contraceptive responsibility are more likely to discuss contraception with their last partner, intent to use, and use contraception (Pleck et al., 1990, 1991; Marsiglio, 1993). Males with more traditional beliefs about men's roles are more likely to use contraceptives less (Marsiglio, 1993).

STRATEGIES FOR INTERVENTION

Based on the above descriptions of males in terms of their sexual behavior, contraceptive behavior, risk-taking behavior, and masculinity beliefs, an assessment is suggested. This provides a screening for those who may be at risk for contraceptive nonuse.

Risk assessment for ineffective contraceptive use for males:

- young age
- African American
- in committed or serious relationship
- infrequent sex
- lack of contraception with first sexual experience
- multiple partners
- alcohol or drug use
- low educational aspirations
- beliefs of female contraceptive responsibility
- traditional male role

Several strategies are suggested to facilitate male contraceptive use. First, males' access to services needs to be addressed. Then, once males have access, education, collaborative decision making, and facilitation of communication skills is suggested.

ACCESS TO SERVICES

Innovative and user friendly contraceptive services for males are advocated. It has been noted that there are minimal services (Swanson et al., 1990), low utilization of services, numerous barriers to services (Swanson & Forrest, 1987), and a need for educational resources for males (Forrest, Swanson, & Beckstein, 1989).

Decreasing barriers to services is suggested. Males have noted that clinics are female oriented, have long waiting times, and inconvenient hours (Swanson, 1980); more evening and weekend clinic hours could be made available. Accessing men in the community (such as when making newborn home visits) and referring them to family planning clinics is advocated (Swanson et al., 1990).

Another approach would be to broaden counseling beyond the individual. Couple counseling is advocated (Swanson, 1985) and is appropriate as partners are a contraceptive information source for some men (Swanson, 1980). Facilitating parent and adolescent communication is advocated as parents are a contraceptive information source for some adolescents (Clark et al., 1984). This is an area of concern as adolescent males are less likely than females to discuss sex and contraception with parents (Leland & Barth, 1992).

EDUCATION

Education about contraceptive use is advocated. Information needs to be provided on how to use contraceptives consistently and correctly to be effective in preventing unintended pregnancies, STDs, and HIV. There may be different reasons for using contraceptives. For example, condoms are used for both prevention of pregnancy and STDs by the majority of adult (Glasser et al., 1989) and adolescent males (Orr & Langefeld, 1993). Cultural differences may exist. For example, condoms were used primarily for prevention of STDs and HIV by Hispanic males (Forrest et al., 1993).

Education is especially needed for adolescents who have relatively low levels of sexual and contraceptive knowledge. For example, a considerable portion of African American adolescent males were not knowledgeable about when pregnancy risk was greatest within the female cycle (Clark et al., 1984), about the risk of pregnancy when using withdrawal, nor about protection from spermicides (Jemmott & Jemmott, 1990). However, adolescent males are more knowledgeable about condoms and STD prevention than females (Leland & Barth, 1992).

Education about specific contraceptives is needed. For example, information about vasectomies may include procedural information about having a vasectomy (length of operation, cost, location of incision) and sensory information about having a vasectomy (pain) (Mumford, 1983).

Currently used information sources could be used to provide additional information. Informational brochures could be made available at drugstores and at public health departments, which are sources for obtaining condoms (Glasser et al., 1989). This would be an appropriate medium as reading materials are a contraceptive information source for some males (Clark et al., 1984; Freeman et al., 1980). Other potential sources are school-based clinics and their education programs. Schools are a source of contraceptive information of some males (Freeman et al., 1980). Contraceptive use was greater for high school students who visited a school-based clinic (Galavotti & Lovick, 1989) and whose school-based clinic had an AIDS educational program (Kirby, Waszak, & Ziegler, 1991).

Another approach is directly mailing information to the home. Direct mailing of condom information positively influenced adolescent males' contraceptive knowledge, beliefs, sexual behavior, and ordering of condoms (Kirby et al., 1989).

Training of peers as educators is another approach. Friends are a source of contraceptive information for some males (Clark et al., 1984; Freeman et al., 1980). This is important for men who are considering vasectomies, because discussion with other men who have had a vasectomy is beneficial (Mumford, 1983).

DECISION MAKING

In addition to education, collaborative contraceptive decision making is suggested. Collaboration may involve beliefs related to specific contraceptive methods, risk taking, and masculinity. Beliefs provide a focus for discussion to facilitate contraceptive decision making and use (see Chapter 3). Male contraceptive use is associated with more positive contraceptive attitudes (Ewald & Roberts, 1985; Jemmott & Jemmott, 1990; Orr & Langefeld, 1993) and beliefs (Joffe & Radius, 1993; Kegeles, Adler, & Irwin, 1989; Pleck et al., 1990, 1993; Tanfer et al., 1993).

There is some information on males' contraceptive beliefs (see Table 5.5). Some of these beliefs are similar to reasons for not using contraceptives such as embarrassment (Reis et al., 1987), discomfort (Reis et al., 1987), and the nature of sex changes (Forrest et al., 1993).

The favorableness of one method over another may be related to reversibility of the method and user's age. It may be that those who wish to delay parenthood are more likely to favor temporary methods. For example, young men view condoms favorably (Pleck et al., 1991) and rate oral contraceptives, condoms, and diaphragms the highest among 13 methods (McDermott et al., 1993). In contrast, men who have decided to have no more children view vasectomies favorably (Mumford, 1983).

Males' contraceptive attitudes differ from females'. Young males are more favorable toward condoms (Norris & Ford, 1994) and have greater perceived self-confidence in their ability to buy and use condoms correctly than females (Kasen, Vaughan, & Walter, 1992).

TABLE 5.5. **Perceptions of Contraceptives**

Perceived benefits	Perceived barriers
Beliefs about contraception	
Prevent pregnancy	Messy
	Less enjoyment
	Not natural
	Harmful for partner's body
Beliefs about vasectomy	
Effective	Painful procedure
Lack of side effects	Inconvenience of having
No interference with sexual pleasure	operation
Beliefs about condoms	
Effective	Embarrassment
Able to have sex at spur of moment	Diminished pleasure
Easy to use	Alters nature of sex
Popular with peers	Must withdraw right away
Makes man responsible for birth control	Uncomfortable
Partner appreciates condom use	Need to be careful or will break
Partner wants condom used	Infers unfaithfulness
Shows you are a caring person	Girls won't want you to use

Sources: Clark et al. (1984); Forrest et al. (1993); Grady et al. (1993); Jemmott & Jemmott (1990); Kegeles et al. (1988, 1989); Mumford (1983); Pleck et al. (1990, 1993); and Swanson (1980).

COMMUNICATION

Facilitating communication with partners about contraceptives is suggested. Males' contraceptive use is associated with beliefs about their ability to discuss and actual discussion about contraception (Delamater & Maccorquodale, 1978; Thompson & Spanier, 1978). This is a particular need among adolescent males as fewer than half discussed contraception with their partner (Ku et al., 1993; Marsiglio, 1993).

Facilitation of communication with partners could involve watching a video of others communicating successfully or practicing contraceptive discussions in an hypothetical situation. Practicing a skill and watching the skill of another are proposed to influence one's confidence and ability to perform a skill (Bandura, 1992). This approach is supported by research findings. Watching others and practicing the resistance of social pressure and negotiation of interpersonal situations decreased unprotected sex (Kirby et al., 1991). Practicing communication related to sex and contraception positively influenced communication skills

(Kelly et al., 1989; Solomon & DeJong, 1989) and the use of contraception (Eisen, Zellman, & McAlister, 1990, Kelly et al., 1989; Solomon & DeJong, 1989).

SUMMARY

Assessment of sexual, contraceptive, and risk-taking behavior, as well as masculinity beliefs helps screen for those who may be at risk for contraceptive nonuse. Education, collaborative decision making, and facilitation of communication skills are suggested.

REFERENCES

Anderson, J., Freese, T., & Pennbridge, J. (1994). Sexual risk behavior and condom use among street youth in Hollywood. *Family Planning Perspectives, 26,* 22–25.

Bandura, A. (1992). A social cognitive approach to the exercise of control over AIDS infection. In R. DiClemente (Ed.), *Adolescents and AIDS: A generation in jeopardy* (pp. 89–116). Newbury Park: SAGE.

Billy, J., Tanfer, K., Grady, W., & Klepinger, D. (1993). The sexual behavior of men in the United States. *Family Planning Perspectives, 25,* 52–60.

Biglan, A., Metzler, C., Wirt, R., Ary, D., Noell, J., Ochs, L., French, C., & Hood, D. (1990). Social and behavioral factors associated with high-risk sexual behavior among adolescents. *Journal of Behavioral Medicine, 13,* 245–261.

Catania, J., Coates, T., Kegeles, S., Fullilove, M., Peterson, J., Marin, B., Siegel, D., & Hulley, S. (1992). Condom use in multi-ethnic neighborhoods of San Francisco: The population-based AMEN (AIDS in multi-ethnic neighborhoods) study. *American Journal of Public Health, 82,* 284–287.

Center for Disease Control. (1993). Distribution of STD clinic patients along a stage-of-behavioral-change continuum—selected sites, 1993. *Mortality & Morbidity Weekly Report, 42*(45), 880–883.

Clark, S., Zabin L., & Hardy, J. (1984). Sex, contraception and parenthood: Experience and attitudes among urban Black young men. *Family Planning Perspectives, 16,* 77–82.

Delamater, J., & Maccorquodale, P. (1978). Premarital contraceptive use: A test of two models. *Journal of Marriage & Family, 40,* 235–247.

Eisen, M., Zellman, G., & McAlister, A. (1990). Evaluating the impact of a theory-based sexuality and contraceptive education program. *Family Planning Perspectives, 22*(6), 261–271.

Ewald, B., & Roberts, C. (1985). Contraceptive behavior in college-age males related to Fishbein model. *Advances in Nursing Science, 7*(3), 63–69.

Forrest, K., Austin, D., Valdes, M., Fuentes, E., & Wilson, S. (1993). Exploring norms and beliefs related to AIDS prevention among California Hispanic men. *Family Planning Perspectives, 25,* 111–117.

Forrest, K., Swanson, J., & Beckstein, D. (1989). The availability of educational and training materials on men's reproductive health. *Family Planning Perspectives, 21,* 120–122.

Freeman, E., Rickels, K., Huggins, G., Mudd, E., Garcia, C., & Dickens, H. (1980). Adolescent contraceptive use: Comparison of male and female attitudes and information. *American Journal of Public Health, 70,* 790–797.

Gallen, M., Liskin, L., & Kak, N. (1986). Men—New focus for family planning programs. *Population Reports, 14,* 889–919.

Galavotti, C., & Lovick, S. (1989). School-based clinic use and other factors affecting adolescent contraceptive behavior. *Journal of Adolescent Health Care, 10,* 506–512.

Glasser, M., Dennis, J., Orthoefer, J., Carter, S., & Hollander, E. (1989). Characteristics of males at a public health department contraceptive service. *Journal of Adolescent Health Care, 10,* 115–118.

Gold, D., & Berger, C. (1983). The influence of psychological and situational factors on the contraceptive behavior of single men: A review of the literature. *Population & Environment, 6,* 113–129.

Grady, W., Klepinger, D., Billy, J., & Tanfer, K. (1993). Condom characteristics: The perception and preferences of men in the United States. *Family Planning Perspectives, 25,* 67–73.

Hingson, R., Strunin, L., Berlin, B., & Heeren, T. (1990). Beliefs about AIDS, use of alcohol and drugs, and unprotected sex among Massachusetts adolescents. *American Journal of Public Health, 80,* 295–299.

Jemmott, J., & Jemmott, L. (1993). Alcohol and drug use during sexual activity: Predicting HIV-risk related behaviors of inner-city black male adolescents. *Journal of Adolescent Research, 8,* 41–57.

Jemmott, L., & Jemmott, J. (1990). Sexual knowledge, attitudes, and risky sexual behavior among inner-city black male adolescents. *Journal of Adolescent Research, 5,* 346–369.

Joffe, A., & Radius, S. (1993). Self-efficacy and intent to use condoms among entering college freshman. *Journal of Adolescent Health, 14,* 262–268.

Kasen S., Vaughan, R., & Walter, H. (1992). Self-efficacy for AIDS preventive behaviors among tenth grade students. *Health Education Quarterly, 19,* 187–202.

Kegeles, S., Adler, N., & Irwin, C. (1989). Adolescents and condoms: Association of beliefs with intentions to use. *American Journal of Disease of Children, 143,* 911–915.

Keller, S., Bartlett, J., Schleifer, S., Johnson, R., Pinner, E., & Delaney, B. (1991). HIV-relevant sexual behavior among a healthy inner-city heterosexual adolescent population in an endemic area of HIV. *Journal of Adolescent Health, 12,* 44–48.

Kelly, J., Lawrence, J., Hood, H., & Brasfield, T. (1989). Behavioral intervention to reduce AIDS risk activities. *Journal of Consulting and Clinical Psychology, 57,* 60–67.

Kirby, D., Barth, R., Leland, N., & Fetro, J. (1991). Reducing the risk: Impact of a new curriculum on sexual risk-taking. *Family Planning Perspectives, 23,* 253–263.

Kirby, D., Harvey, P., Claussenius, D., & Novar, M. (1989). A direct mailing to teenage males about condom use: Its impact on knowledge, attitudes and sexual behavior. *Family Planning Perspectives, 21,* 12–18.

Kirby, D., Waszak, C., & Ziegler, J. (1991). Six school-based clinics: Their reproductive health services and impact on sexual behavior. *Family Planning Perspectives, 23,* 6–13.

Ku, L., Sonenstein, F., & Pleck, J. (1993). Factors influencing first intercourse for teenage men. *Public Health Reports, 108,* 680–694.

Leland, N., & Barth, R. (1992). Gender differences in knowledge, intentions, and behaviors concerning pregnancy and sexually transmitted disease prevention among adolescents. *Journal of Adolescent Health, 13,* 589–599.

Marin, B., Gomez, C., & Hearst, N. (1993). Multiple heterosexual partners and condom use among Hispanic and non-Hispanic whites. *Family Planning Perspectives, 25,* 170–174.

Marsiglio, W. (1988). Adolescent male sexuality and heterosexual masculinity: A conceptual model and review. *Journal of Adolescent Research, 3,* 285–303.

Marsiglio, W. (1993). Adolescent males' orientation toward paternity and contraception. *Family Planning Perspectives, 25,* 22–31.

Maticka-Tyndale, E. (1991). Sexual scripts and AIDS prevention: Variations in adherence to safer-sex guidelines by heterosexual adolescents. *Journal of Sex Research, 28,* 45–66.

McDermott, R., Sarvela, P., Gold, R., Holcomb, D., Huetteman, J., & Odulana, J. (1993). Attributes assigned to contraception by college students: 1985 and 1990. *Health Values, 17,* 33–41.

Mumford, S. (1983). The vasectomy decision-making process. *Studies in Family Planning, 14,* 83–88.

Netting, N. (1992). Sexuality in youth culture: Identity and change. *Adolescence, 27,* 961–976.

Norris, A., & Ford, K. (1994). Condom beliefs in urban, low income, African American and Hispanic Youth. *Health Education Quarterly, 21,* 39–53.

Orr, D., & Langefeld, C. (1993). Factors associated with condom use by sexually active male adolescents at risk for sexually transmitted disease. *Pediatrics, 91,* 873–879.

Pleck, J., Sonenstein, F., & Ku, L. (1990). Contraceptive attitudes and intention to use condoms in sexually experienced and inexperienced adolescent males. *Journal of Family Issues, 11,* 294–312.

Pleck, J., Sonenstein, F., & Ku, L. (1991). Adolescent males' condom use: Relationships between perceived cost-benefits and consistency. *Journal of Marriage & Family, 53,* 733–745.

Pleck, J., Sonenstein, F., & Ku, L. (1993). Changes in adolescent males' use of and attitudes toward condoms, 1988–1991. *Family Planning Perspectives, 25,* 106–109, 117.

Pleck, J., Sonenstein, F., & Swain, S. (1988). Adolescent males' sexual behavior and contraceptive use: Implications for male responsibility. *Journal of Adolescent Research, 3,* 275–284.

Reis, J., Reid, E., Herr, T., & Herz, E. (1987). Family planning for inner-city adolescent males: Pilot Study. *Adolescence, 22,* 953–960.

Solomon, M., & DeJong, W. (1989). Preventing AIDS and other STDs through condom promotion: A patient education intervention. *American Journal of Public Health, 79,* 453–458.

Sonenstein, F., Pleck, F., & Ku, L. (1989). Sexual activity, condom use and AIDS awareness among adolescent males. *Family Planning Perspectives, 21,* 152–158.

Sonenstein, F., Pleck, F., & Ku, L. (1991). Levels of sexual activity among adolescent males in the United States. *Family Planning Perspectives, 23,* 162–167.

Sorenson, R. (1973). *Adolescent sexuality in contemporary America.* New York: World Publishing.

Swanson, J. (1980). Knowledge, knowledge, who's got the knowledge? The male contraceptive career. *Journal of Sex Education & Therapy, 6*(2), 51–57.

Swanson, J. (1985). Men and family planning. In S. Hanson & F. Bozett (Eds.), *Dimensions of Fatherhood* (pp. 21–48). Beverly Hills: SAGE.

Swanson, J., & Forrest, K. (1987). Men's reproductive health services in family planning settings: A pilot study. *American Journal of Public Health, 77,* 1462–1463.

Swanson, J., Swenson, I., Oakley, D., & Marcy, S. (1990). Community health nurses and family planning services for men. *Journal of Community Health Nursing, 7,* 87–96.

Tanfer, K., Grady, W., Klepinger, D., & Billy, J. (1993). Condom use among U.S. men, 1991. *Family Planning Perspectives, 25,* 61–66.

Tanner, J. (1971). Sequence, tempo, and individual variation in growth and development of boys and girls aged 12 to 16. In R. Muuss (Ed.), *Adolescent behavior and society: A book of readings* (pp. 36–52). New York: Random House.

Thomas, S., & Hodges, B. (1991). Assessing AIDS knowledge, attitudes, and risk behaviors among Black and Hispanic homosexual and bisexual men: Results of a feasibility study. *Journal of Sex Education & Therapy, 17,* 116–124.

Thompson, L., & Spanier, G. (1978). Influence of parents, peers, and partners on the contraceptive use of college men and women. *Journal of Marriage & Family, 40,* 481–492.

Zotti, M., & Siegel, E. (1995). Preventing unplanned pregnancies among married couples: Are services for only the wife sufficient? *Research in Nursing and Health, 18,* 133–142.

Female Adolescents: Novice Contraceptors

Kathleen M. Hanna

This chapter discusses a perspective on female adolescents' contraceptive use—novice contraceptors. The focus will be on the influence of contraceptive inexperience as well as development. It is neither the intent to review antecedents to sexual behavior, nor all factors that influence contraceptive use. For reviews, the reader is referred to Morrison (1985) or Whitley and Schofield (1985, 1986). It is also not the intent to address the entire adolescent pregnancy problem.

Adolescent pregnancy is a complex problem and not all adolescents are at risk for pregnancy for the same reasons. Adolescents differ in their background and characteristics, and ultimately in their risk for pregnancy and parenthood. Differences among female adolescents who were successfully using contraceptives, were having abortions, were currently pregnant, and were mothers have been reported. For example, adolescents who were mothers were different from these other groups in that they held more traditional beliefs about a woman's role, perceived others or events to be in control of their lives rather than personal control, and had more difficulty thinking of the future (Resnick & Blum, 1985).

Adolescents who become pregnant and become mothers are noted to be a socially and economically disadvantaged group who tend to be poor, members of minority groups, and from inner cities or rural areas (Geronimus, 1991). It is suggested that these disadvantages contribute to adolescents becoming pregnant and parents, rather than simply leading to disadvantaged lives (Geronimus, 1991). Support for this is in adolescent mothers' descriptions of their prepregnant lives in terms of "inheriting a diminished future" (SmithBattle, 1995).

A considerable portion of female adolescents become pregnant. In the most recently published national data, the 1987 pregnancy rate for 15- to 19-year-old females was 127 out of every 1,000 in the United States (Forrest & Singh, 1990). These statistics need to be placed in perspective. Adolescents who became pregnant are a small portion of the total adolescent population. Further, the outcomes for these pregnancies were 50% live births, 36% abortions, and 14% miscarriages (Forrest & Singh, 1990). These statistics support that not all female adolescents choose to become mothers, with a considerable portion not becoming pregnant. However, it must be acknowledged that a predominant portion of those who gave birth wished to be mothers. Of 15- to 19-year-olds who gave birth, 76.8% reported that the infant was wanted at conception (Williams & Pratt, 1990). These statistics support that there are different subpopulations of adolescents at risk for pregnancy and parenthood.

This chapter addresses facilitating contraceptive use among adolescents who are sexually active, wishing to prevent pregnancy, and seeking contraceptives. The strategies discussed can be implemented in relatively brief interactions during a clinic visit. Strategies other than those delineated in this book are needed to address adolescents who wish to become pregnant and parents, and the reader is referred to Hayes (1987) or Humenick, Wilkerson, and Paul (1991).

FEMALE ADOLESCENTS' SEXUAL AND CONTRACEPTIVE BEHAVIOR

SEXUAL BEHAVIOR

Female adolescents are inexperienced as sexual persons with reproductive capabilities. Maturation of reproductive organs and development of secondary sex characteristics occur with higher levels of estrogen production during puberty (Tanner, 1971). Sexual behavior becomes significant when reproduction is possible.

Based on national surveys in the United States and Canada, female adolescents' typical sexual behavior can be described (see Table 6.1)—approximately half have had sexual intercourse. The incidence of having had sexual intercourse increases with age.

TABLE 6.1. Percentage of Female Adolescents Who Have Had Sexual Intercourse at Least Once by Years of Age for Various Years

Age	United States					Canada
	1971	1976	1979	1982	1988	1976
15	15	19	23	17		8
16	22	30	40	29		
17	28	46	50	41		
16–17						19
18	43	57	63	59		
19	48	64	71	72		
15–19	30	43	50	45	53	
18–23						60

Note: United States data sources were Hofferth, Kahn, and Baldwin (1987) for unmarried females in 1971 and 1982 and Forrest and Singh (1990) for married and unmarried females in 1988. Canadian data source was Jones et al. (1986) for married and unmarried females in 1976. When comparing the rates, it should be noted that data are reported for different years, age groups, marital status, and questions to measure sexual behavior.

Infrequent sexual intercourse and serial monogamy are typical for female adolescents. The majority (60%) of 15- to 19-year-old females have had sexual intercourse as infrequently as 0 to 3 times a month in 1982 (Hofferth & Hayes, 1987). Serial monogamy, a sexual relationship with only one person for an uncertain length of time, has been the most common type of sexual relationship among adolescents (Netting, 1992; Sorenson, 1973). The majority (60%) of 15- to 19-year-old females were in a serious relationship—engaged or going steady—with their initial sexual partner (Zelnik, 1983). However, this relationship obviously was not permanent as 58% of 15- to 19-year-old females have had sexual intercourse with 2 or more partners in their lifetime (Forrest & Singh, 1990).

CONTRACEPTIVE BEHAVIOR

Based on national surveys of female adolescents in the United States and Canada, contraceptive behavior can be described (see Table 6.2). Contraceptive use has been relatively low; however, it has been increasing. In the United States, approximately one-third used contraceptives. In Canada, half (a slightly older sample than the United States) used contraceptives. The oral contraceptive pill was the most frequently

TABLE 6.2.   Percentages for Various Methods
for Canadian and United States' Female
Adolescents Who Use Contraceptives

	United States		Canada
Year	1982	1988	1984
Contraceptive method			
Any method	24	32	50
Condom	21	33	9
Pill	64	59	84
Diaphragm	6	1	0
IUD	1	0	1

Note: Source for 15- to 19-year-old married and unmarried females
in the United States is Mosher (1990), and for 18- to 19-year-old
married and unmarried females in Canada is Jones et al. (1986).
When comparing the rates, it should be noted that data are reported for different years, age groups, and marital status.

used method by those who used contraceptives. However, the use of oral
contraceptives has decreased recently while condom use has increased.

CONTRACEPTIVE ADHERENCE

Although female adolescents' contraceptive adherence may be described,
the data are not from nationally representative samples. Adherence varied between 10% and 70% for various methods (see Table 6.3).
Adherence was greater for those who were older. On the average, 2.7
to 3.4 oral contraceptive pills per month were not taken because they
were forgotten (Balassone, 1989). Condom use with the pill was very
low and was lower for those who have one sexual partner than for
those who have single, short-term sexual partners. Examples of reasons for nonadherence included not currently being sexually active,
forgetting to take the pill, and concern about the side effects of contraception (Delmore, Kalagian, & Loewen, 1991).

SUMMARY

The data presented provide a description of typical female adolescents' contraceptive and sexual behavior. However, sexual and contraceptive behavior may differ from nationally representative samples for
female adolescents in specific regions, communities, or settings.

TABLE 6.3. Female Adolescents' Rates of Adherence to Contraceptives

Study	Contraceptive and measurement method	Age in years	Rate (%)
Litt et al. (1980)	Kept appointment and self-reported use of pill, IUD, diaphragm, and no pregnancy	12–15 16–21	37 63
Freeman et al. (1982)	Self-reported "always" used pill, condom, or diaphragm	12–17	62
Scher et al. (1982)	No interruption in pill regimen by self-report and chart review	14–25	62
Neel et al. (1985)	No pregnancy and pill use by self-report and serum/urine levels	M = 16 M = 20	48 70
Balassone (1989)	Appointment-keeping	M = 16	55
Weisman et al. (1991)	Consistent pill use when were: * consistent condom user * inconsistent condom user Consistent condom use when had: * single, stable partner * single, short-term partner * multiple partner Consistent pill and condom user	11–18	 25 41 14 24 10 12
Hanna (1990)	Pill taking with no missed days kept appointment	16–18	61 67
Kegeles et al. (1989)	Used condoms every time	14–19	2
Rickert et al. (1989)	Used condoms with other contraception	12–19	10
DiClemente et al. (1992)	Always used condoms	7–9th graders	44

Note: Comparisons between studies should be done cautiously when contraceptive adherence has been operationally defined and measured by various means (Beck & Davis, 1987; Whitley and Schofield, 1985, 1986).

PROCESS OF CHOOSING AND USING CONTRACEPTIVES

Contraceptive use among female adolescents and young adults has been described as a process (Lindeman, 1974). The process involves three stages: the natural stage (nonuse of contraception), the peer stage (use of nonprescription contraception), and the expert stage (use of prescription contraception). This process is supported by a meta-analysis of research findings on adolescent contraceptive use (Whitley & Schofield, 1985, 1986).

NATURAL STAGE

According to Lindeman (1974), female adolescents and young adults who are initiating sexual behavior are in the natural stage. Sexual behavior is unpredictable, infrequent, and not integrated into one's self-concept; therefore, there is indecision about sexual activity and failure to seek contraceptives. The natural stage is supported by adolescent developmental theory and research findings, especially for very young adolescents.

Contraceptive use has been low for young female adolescents who were beginning to be sexually active. The majority did not use contraception with first sexual intercourse (see Table 6.4). However, the portion has been increasing due to an increased use of condoms. Contraceptive nonuse was greater for young females who were beginners with fewer years postmenarche (DuRant & Sanders, 1989), fewer years dating (DuRant & Sanders, 1989), fewer years having had sexual intercourse (DuRant & Sanders, 1989), and less frequent sexual intercourse (DuRant & Sanders, 1989; Whitley & Schofield, 1985, 1986).

Young female adolescents who are beginning sexual activity most likely have not integrated their sexual self into their identity. During

TABLE 6.4.   Percentages of Female Adolescents Using Contraceptive Methods at First Sexual Intercourse

Contraception	15–19 1982	15–19 1988	< 14	15–16	17–18	> 19
No method used	52	35	61	53	46	44
Any method used	48	65	39	47	54	56
Methods used:						
Condom	23	47	23	29	30	24
Pill	8	8	6	8	12	18
Withdrawal	13	8	9	9	8	8
Other	4	< 1	2	1	4	6

Note: Source for 1982 to 1988 data for married and unmarried females is Forrest and Singh (1990). Source for data for various ages of unmarried females in 1988 is Mosher and McNally (1990). When comparing the rates, it should be noted that data are reported for different years and age groups.

the developmental period of adolescence, adolescents are in the process of consolidating their psychological identities (Erikson, 1968), that is, integrating past (being a nonsexual person), present (beginning to be a sexual person), and future (being a sexual person).

Sexual self-acceptance is most likely associated with integration of the sexual self into one's identity. Contraceptive nonuse was greater for those who lack sexual self-acceptance (Whitley & Schofield, 1985, 1986). Lack of sexual self-acceptance was suggested in that only a minority of adolescent couples (28%) discussed contraception prior to first sexual intercourse (Polit-O'Hara & Kahn, 1985).

Female adolescents' lack of sexual self-acceptance may be related to inconsistent beliefs. Inconsistencies in beliefs that sex is bad and pleasurable need to be resolved (Kagan, 1971). Contraceptive use would mean that sexual intercourse was planned, and as Fox (1977) noted "nice girls don't plan for sex." Contraceptives nonuse was greater for adolescents who did not plan to have sexual intercourse (Whitley & Schofield, 1985, 1986).

The natural stage is further supported by female adolescents' lack of sexual and contraceptive knowledge. One (Morrison, 1985; Scott et al., 1988) to four contraceptive methods (Herz, Goldberg, & Reis, 1984) have been identified by adolescents. However, many have insufficient knowledge on how contraception prevents pregnancy (Scott et al., 1988). Knowledge of fertility and reproduction was limited with fewer than half having accurate knowledge of the life expectancy of the sperm (Lowe & Radius, 1987; Morrison, 1985) and of the risk of pregnancy within the menstrual cycle (Lowe & Radius, 1987; Morrison, 1985; Reschovsky & Gerner, 1991).

PEER PRESCRIPTION STAGE

Next is the peer prescription stage where female adolescents and young adults explore and experiment with sexual behavior and contraception. Acknowledgement of their sexual self to themselves and their sexual partners begins. However, acknowledgement of their sexual self to parents or professionals is feared. Therefore, prescription contraceptive methods are not sought, but experimentation with nonprescription methods such as condoms, withdrawal, foam, douches, and rhythm occurs. The peer stage is supported in that the condom, a nonprescription method, was used with first sexual intercourse by slightly fewer than half (see Table 6.4). Additionally, condoms were the predominant method for young females.

The peer stage is further supported in the area of female adolescents' relationships with friends and partners. Reliance on peers is important as adolescents lessen their dependence upon parents in becoming independent and responsible adults (Blos, 1979). Adolescents' dependence on peers in the area of contraception is supported in that the majority discussed contraception with friends and partners (Herold & Samson, 1980; Delmore et al., 1991), and specifically since their first sexual intercourse experience (Polit-O'Hara & Kahn, 1985). Friends were the most frequent source of contraceptive information (Delmore et al., 1991; Milan & Kilmann, 1987; Morrison, 1985) and greatest source of contraceptive support (Delmore et al., 1991).

In contrast to adolescents' discussion about contraceptives with peers, adolescents do not acknowledge their sexual self to parents. Adolescents are developing psychological identities as separate and independent persons from their parents (Blos, 1979). Adolescents who are striving to have their own unique identity that is separate from their parents may need to keep their sexual self private until their identity is more firmly established.

Support exists for the relationship between female adolescents' contraceptive nonuse and fear of acknowledgement of their sexual self to parents. Only a minority communicated with parents about sexual matters (Demetriou & Kaplan, 1989) and contraception (Morrison, 1985). Parents were the least frequent source of contraceptive information (Milan & Kilmann, 1987; Morrison, 1985). A frequent reason for contraceptive nonuse was concern about parental reaction to sexual and contraceptive behavior (Whitley & Schofield, 1985, 1986; Zabin, Stark & Emerson, 1991). Fear of parents' anger was a concern when seeking contraceptives (Demetriou & Kaplan, 1989).

EXPERT STAGE

During Lindeman's (1974) expert stage, female adolescents and young adults acknowledge their sexual self and seek contraceptives from professionals. Sexual self-acceptance is influenced by frequent sexual intercourse within a committed close relationship.

Female adolescents in this stage are more likely to be older, to have been sexually active for awhile, and to be using contraceptives. Contraceptive use was greater for older female adolescents (Mosher & McNally, 1991), with more frequent sexual intercourse (DuRant, Jay, & Seymore, 1990; DuRant & Sanders, 1989; DuRant et al., 1988; Litt, Cuskey, & Rudd, 1980; Whitley & Schofield, 1985, 1986), with greater number of years of sexual activity (DuRant & Sanders, 1989), with greater number of years of dating (DuRant & Sanders, 1989), with previous contraceptive use (Delmore et al., 1991; DuRant et al., 1988), with a single sexual partner (DuRant et al., 1984; Litt et al., 1980), and within a close relationship with a sexual partner (Whitley & Schofield, 1985, 1986).

These older female adolescents would be more likely to accept their sexual self and to plan for sexual intercourse. The planning for sexual intercourse is supported in that contraceptive use was greater for those who initiate intercourse at an older age (see Table 6.4). Contraceptive use was associated with planning for sexual intercourse, acceptance of sexual self (Whitley & Schofield, 1985, 1986), and a positive sexual self-concept (Winter, 1988).

Female adolescents who accept their sexuality most likely communicate with parents and peers about contraceptives. Contraceptive use was greater for those who communicated with partners (Loewenstein & Furstenberg, 1991), parents (Campbell & Barnlund, 1977), parents about sexual matters (Demetriou & Kaplan, 1989; Loewenstein & Furstenberg, 1991; Reschovsky & Gerner, 1991), parents about contraceptives (Casper, 1990), and with mothers about contraceptives (Fox & Inazu, 1980; Herold & Samson, 1980; Newcomer & Udry, 1985).

The expert stage is further supported by the change from less effective to more effective contraceptives. A considerable number of female adolescents switched from a nonmedical to a medical contraceptive method (Hirsch & Zelnik, 1985). An effective, prescription method— the oral contraceptive pill—becomes a more predominant method for older females (see Table 6.4).

The long duration between initiation of sexual intercourse and seeking prescription methods further supports the expert stage. Among various samples of female adolescents, the average interval between initiating sexual intercourse experience and seeking of contraceptives from health professionals varied from 12 to 17 months (Balassone, 1989; Zabin & Clark, 1981; Zabin et al., 1991; Zelnik, Koenig, & Kim, 1984). Contraceptive use was negatively associated with length of time between initiating sex and seeking contraceptives (DuRant et al., 1988).

SUMMARY

This description of female adolescents' process of using contraceptives provides an understanding of their contraceptive behavior. Inexperienced female adolescents in the natural and peer prescription stages of the process are most likely at the greatest risk for nonuse or ineffective use of contraceptives. Based on this description, those at risk for contraceptive nonuse or ineffective use may be identified.

CONTRACEPTIVE DECISION MAKING
OR PROBLEM SOLVING

Female adolescents' contraceptive behavior may be further explained by their inexperience in contraceptive decision making and problem solving. Inexperienced contraceptive decision makers–problem solvers may not consider the consequences of contraception—perceived benefits and barriers to contraception—nor address the negative consequences of contraception—perceived contraceptive barriers. See Chapter 3 for a review of contraceptive decision making and problem solving.

CONTRACEPTIVE PERCEPTIONS

Female adolescents' contraceptive perceptions—elements of contraceptive decision making and problem solving—provides a means to understand and predict contraceptive use. Examples of adolescents' perceptions of susceptibility of pregnancy, seriousness of pregnancy and parenthood, and barriers and benefits of contraception are outlined in Table 6.5. Contraceptive perceptions have influenced contraceptive use (see Chapter 3).

Strategies are advocated that involve promoting adolescents' contraceptive decision making and problem solving, and ultimately contraceptive use. Contraceptive decision making and problem solving can be improved with contraceptive knowledge and experience.

Contraceptive education is warranted for insufficient contraceptive knowledge. Support exists for the influence of education on contraceptive use (see Chapter 3). Some hold the belief that education promotes sexual behavior. However, provision of sexual and contraceptive knowledge did not influence initiation of sexual behavior (Eisen & Zellman, 1987; Kirby, Waszak, & Ziegler, 1991), or frequency of sex (Kirby et al., 1991). Sexual and contraceptive knowledge needs to be assessed and addressed. Female adolescents who are beginning to initiate sexual and contraceptive behavior most likely have insufficient contraceptive knowledge. Although contraceptive education is needed, it is not sufficient.

In addition to education, facilitation of contraceptive decision making and problem solving as discussed in Chapter 3 is suggested. Adherence to oral contraceptives was greater among female adolescents who had identified their contraceptive perceptions and explored means to diminish contraceptive barriers with nurses than those who had not (Hanna, 1993).

TABLE 6.5. Female Adolescents' Contraceptive Perceptions

Benefits	Barriers

Contraception in general

Benefits	Barriers
Prevention of pregnancy	Against religious beliefs
Self-responsibility	Embarrassment
Control of one's life	Planning for sex
Partner more willing	Ineffectiveness
to have sex	Trouble
Partner will know care	Side effects
Partner will know smart	Dirty
Improves relationship	Uncomfortable
Feel more like an adult	Important to take chance to show love

Oral contraceptives

Benefits	Barriers
Prevention of pregnancy	Harmful health effects
Self-responsibility	Side effects
Approval by others	Disapproval by others

Condoms

Benefits	Barriers
Spontaneous sex possible	Harmful health effects
Easy to use	Difficult to use
Self-responsibility	Planning for sex
Protection from STDs	Uncomfortable to use
Sex lasts longer	Feel guilty
Neatness	Break the mood
Sex more exciting	Unreliable
Show concern and caring	Messy
Sex more pleasurable	Sex doesn't feel right and less
Safe	pleasurable
Prevents pregnancy	Interrupts sex
	Sex less romantic
	Inconvenient
	Partner will think you are having sex
	with others
	Partner will think you don't trust him

Sources: Brown (1984), Eisen et al. (1985), Hanna (1994), Kalmuss et al. (1987), Kegeles et al. (1989), Norris & Ford (1994), and Scott et al. (1988).

INFLUENCE OF DEVELOPMENT OF CONTRACEPTIVE PERCEPTIONS

Egocentrism, an aspect of adolescents' cognitive development, may help explain some contraceptive perceptions. Adolescents may perceive themselves as unique according to the "personal fable" described by Elkind (1967). Low perceived susceptibility to pregnancy may reflect perceptions of uniqueness in terms of invulnerability to pregnancy. Adolescents may also think others are thinking the same thoughts as they are according to the "imaginary audience" described by Elkind (1967). These adolescents may be concerned that others may see them obtain and use contraceptives—perceived contraceptive barriers. Adolescents' egocentric thinking has been reported to limit contraceptive problem solving (Green, Johnson, & Kaplan, 1992).

Cognitive functioning may influence contraceptive perceptions and decision making and problem solving. Adolescents' low levels of perceived susceptibility to pregnancy may be explained by cognitively processing inaccurate information. Many overestimated their probability of becoming pregnant (Lowe & Radius, 1987; Morrison, 1985). Morrison (1985) suggested that this overestimation leads adolescents to judge themselves infertile after having had sexual intercourse without becoming pregnant. They are processing what information they have; however, they may be lacking information on reproductive ability. Menstrual periods may be anovulatory for up to 18 months post menarche (Tanner, 1971). Cognitive functioning may also be influenced by contraceptive inexperience (see Chapter 3).

Contraceptive perceptions may be influenced by psychosocial development within families. Adolescents seek to achieve psychological identities as separate and autonomous persons from parents (Blos, 1979; Erikson, 1968). In this process, adolescents renegotiate relationships with parents and become more independent and self-responsible. While lessening dependence upon parents, peers are relied upon. Contraceptive use may be influenced by parents and/or peers. Intention to use and actual use of contraceptives were influenced by: parents (Baker, Thalberg, & Morrison, 1988; Jorgensen & Sonstegard, 1984), expectations of others (Adler, Kegeles, Irwin, & Wibbeisman, 1990), mothers' approval of sex (White, 1987), and partners (Weisman, Plichta, Nathanson, Ensminger, & Robinson, 1991; Whitley & Schofield, 1985, 1986). Who is influential may be related to the quality of relationship with parents. Adolescents who perceived parents' sexual and contraceptive communication as more caring have greater use of contraceptives than adolescents who perceive parents' communication as "contentious" and "dramatic" (Mueller & Powers, 1990).

These relationships may be helpful to the adolescent in terms of seeking contraceptive information and receiving support for contraception. This information may be assessed by the health care professional during the clinic visit and used in promoting contraceptive use. For example, if friends are identified as a source of support, they may be encouraged to provide contraceptive support such as accompaniment to a clinic. Peers have been used to provide contraceptive care and this care has positively influenced contraceptive use (Jay et al., 1984). If self-reliance is evident, contraceptive use may be promoted by working independently with the adolescent, since those who seek contraception have a relatively high level of autonomy in relation to parents (Hanna, 1990).

In summary, a list of questions that would aid in the assessment of adolescents' contraceptive behavior related to seeking and receiving support would include:

1. Who are information sources for sex and contraception?
2. Who was involved in the decision to use contraception?
3. With whom has the adolescent discussed contraception?
4. Who made the appointment to get contraception?
5. Who accompanied the adolescent to the clinic or pharmacy?
6. Who helps the adolescent to remember to use contraception?
7. Who helps remember appointments for contraception?
8. Who is responsible for obtaining and using contraception?

CONCLUSIONS

Female adolescents are at risk for unplanned and unwanted pregnancies due to sexual and contraceptive inexperience. In addition, female adolescents are at risk for sexually transmitted diseases (STDs), especially human immunodeficiency virus (HIV). A portion of acquired immunodeficiency syndrome (AIDS) cases in young adulthood may be attributed to the transmission of HIV during adolescence (DiClemente, 1992).

As inexperienced contraceptors, female adolescents' contraceptive use may be promoted through provision of contraceptive information and facilitation of contraceptive decision making and problem solving. Education is necessary, but alone is not sufficient. Promotion of contraceptive decision making and problem solving for prevention of sexually transmitted diseases as well as prevention of pregnancy is also needed. Condom use to prevent sexually transmitted diseases should be advocated along with the choice of a contraceptive method to prevent pregnancy.

REFERENCES

Adler, N., Kegeles, S., Irwin, C., & Wibbeisman, C. (1990). Adolescent contraceptive behavior: An assessment of decision processes. *Journal of Pediatrics, 116,* 463–471.

Baker, S., Thalberg, S., & Morrison, D. (1988). Parents' behavioral norms as predictors of adolescent sexual activity and contraceptive use. *Adolescence, 23,* 265–282.

Balassone, M. (1989). Risk of contraceptive discontinuation among adolescents. *Journal of Adolescent Health Care, 10,* 527–533.

Beck, J., & Davis, D. (1987). Teen contraception: A review of perspectives on compliance. *Archives of Sexual Behavior, 16,* 337–368.

Blos, P. (1979). The second individuation process of adolescence. In P. Blos (Ed.), *The adolescent passage* (pp. 141–170). New York: International Universities Press.

Brown, I. (1984). Development of a scale to measure attitude toward the condom as a method of birth control. *The Journal of Sex Research, 20,* 255–263.

Campbell, B., & Barnlund, D. (1977). Communication patterns and problems of pregnancy. *American Journal of Orthopsychiatry, 47,* 134–139.

Casper, L. (1990). Does family interaction prevent adolescent pregnancy? *Family Planning Perspectives, 22,* 109–114.

Delmore, T., Kalagian, W., & Loewen, I. (1991). Follow-up of adolescent oral contraceptive users. *Canadian Journal of Public Health, 82,* 277–278.

Demetriou, E., & Kaplan, D. (1989). Adolescent contraceptive use and parental notification. *American Journal of Diseases of Children, 143,* 1166–1172.

DiClemente, R. (1992). Epidemiology of AIDS, HIV prevalence, and HIV incidence among adolescents. *Journal of School Health, 62,* 325–330.

DuRant, R., Jay, S., Linder, C., Shoffitt, T., & Litt, J. (1984). Influence of psychosocial factors on adolescents' compliance with oral contraceptives. *Journal of Adolescent Health Care, 5,* 1–6.

DuRant, R., Jay, S., & Seymore, C. (1990). Contraceptive and sexual behavior of black female adolescents. *Journal of Adolescent Health Care, 11,* 326–334.

DuRant, R., Sanders, J., Jay, S., & Levinson, R. (1988). Analysis of contraceptive behavior of sexually active female adolescents in the United States. *Journal of Pediatrics, 113,* 930–936.

DuRant, R., & Sanders, J. (1989). Sexual behavior and contraceptive risk taking among sexually active adolescent females. *Journal of Adolescent Health Care, 10,* 1–9.

Eisen, M., Zellman, G., & McAlister, A. (1985). A Health Belief Model approach to adolescents' fertility control: Some pilot program findings. *Health Education Quarterly, 12,* 185–210.

Eisen, M., & Zellman, G. (1987). Changes in incidence of sexual intercourse of unmarried teenagers following a community-based sex education program. *The Journal of Sex Research, 23,* 527–533.

Elkind, D. (1967). Egocentrism in adolescence. *Child Development, 38,* 1025–1034.

Erikson, E. (1968). *Identity: Youth and crisis.* New York: W. W. Norton.

Forrest, J., & Singh, S. (1990). The sexual and reproductive behavior of American women, 1982–1988. *Family Planning Perspectives, 22,* 206–214.

Fox, G. (1977). "Nice girls": Social control of women through a value construct. *SIGNS: Journal of Women in Culture and Society, 2,* 805–817.

Fox, G., & Inazu, J. (1980). Patterns and outcomes of mother-daughter communication about sexuality. *Journal of Social Issues, 36,* 7–29.

Freeman, E., Rickels, K., Mudd, E., & Huggins, G. (1982). Never-pregnant adolescents and family planning programs: Contraception, continuation, and pregnancy risk. *American Journal of Public Health, 72,* 815–822.

Geronimus, A. (1991). Teenage childbearing and social and reproductive disadvantage: The evolution of complex questions and the demise of simple answers. *Family Relations, 40,* 463–471.

Green, V., Johnson, S., & Kaplan, D. (1992). Predictors of adolescent female decision making regarding contraceptive usage. *Adolescence, 27,* 613–631.

Hanna, K. (1990). Effect of nurse-client transaction on female adolescents' contraceptive perceptions and adherence. *Dissertations Abstracts International,* University of Pittsburgh.

Hanna, K. (1993). Effect of nurse-client transaction on female adolescents' oral contraceptive adherence. *IMAGE: Journal of Nursing Scholarship, 25,* 285–290.

Hanna, K. (1994). Female adolescents' perceived benefits and barriers to using oral contraceptives. *Issues in Comprehensive Pediatric Nursing, 17,* 47–55.

Herold, E., & Sampson, L. (1980). Differences between women who begin pill use before and after first intercourse: Ontario, Canada. *Family Planning Perspectives, 12,* 304–305.

Herz, E., Goldberg, W., & Reis, J. (1984). Family life education for young adolescents: A quasi-experiment. *Journal of Youth & Adolescence, 13,* 309–327.

Hirsch, M., & Zelnik, M. (1985). Contraceptive method switching among

American female adolescents, 1979. *Journal of Adolescent Health Care, 6,* 1–7.

Hofferth, S., & Hayes, C. (1987). *Risking the future: Adolescent sexuality, pregnancy, and childbearing; Vol 2.* Washington DC: National Academy Press.

Hofferth, S., Kahn, J., & Baldwin, W. (1987). Premarital sexual activity among U.S. teenage women over the past three decades. *Family Planning Perspectives, 19,* 46–53.

Humenick, S., Wilkerson, N., & Paul, N. (1991). *Adolescent pregnancy: Nursing perspectives on prevention.* White Plains, NY: March of Dimes Birth Defects Foundation.

Jay, S., DuRant, R., Shoffitt, T., Linder, C., & Litt, I. (1984). Effect of peer counselors on adolescents' compliance in use of oral contraceptives. *Pediatrics, 73,* 126–131.

Jones, E., Forrest, J., Goldman, N., Henshaw, S., Lincoln, R., Rosoff, J., Westoff, C., & Wulf, D. (1986). *Teenage Pregnancy in Industrialized Countries.* New Haven: Yale University Press.

Jorgensen, S., & Sonstegard, J. (1984). Predicting adolescent sexual behavior: An application and test of the Fishbein Model. *Journal of Marriage and the Family,* (Feb.), 43–55.

Kagan, J. (1971). A conception of early adolescence. *Daedalus, 100,* 997–1012.

Kalmuss, D., Lawton, A., & Namerow, P. (1987). Advantages and disadvantages of pregnancy and contraception: Teenagers' perceptions. *Population and Environment, 9,* 23–40.

Kegeles, S., Adler, N., & Irwin, C. (1989). Adolescents and condoms: Association of beliefs with intentions to use. *American Journal of Diseases of Children, 143,* 911–915.

Kirby, D., Waszak, C., & Ziegler, J. (1991). Six school-based clinics: Their reproductive health services and impact on sexual behavior. *Family Planning Perspectives, 23,* 6–13.

Lindeman, C. (1974). *Birth Control and Unmarried Young Women.* New York: Springer Publishing.

Litt, I., Cuskey, W., & Rudd, S. (1980). Identifying adolescents at risk for noncompliance with contraceptive therapy. *The Journal of Pediatrics, 96,* 742–745.

Loewenstein, G., & Furstenberg, F. (1991). Is teenage sexual behavior rational? *Journal of Applied Social Psychology, 21,* 957–986.

Lowe, C., & Radius, S. (1987). Young adults' contraceptive practices: An investigation of influences. *Adolescence, 22,* 291–303.

Milan, R., & Kilmann, P. (1987). Interpersonal factors in premarital contraception. *The Journal of Sex Research, 23,* 289–321.

Morrison, D. (1985). Adolescent contraceptive behavior: A review. *Psychology Bulletin, 98,* 538–568.

Mosher, W. (1990). Contraceptive practice in the United States, 1982–1988. *Family Planning Perspectives, 22,* 198–205.

Mosher, W., & McNally, J. (1991). Contraceptive use at first premarital intercourse: United States, 1965–1988. *Family Planning Perspectives, 23,* 108–116.

Mueller, D., & Powers, W. (1990). Parent-child discussion: Perceived communicator style and subsequent behavior. *Adolescence, 25,* 469–482.

Neel, E., Jay, S., & Litt, I. (1985). The relationship of self-concept and autonomy to oral contraceptive compliance among adolescent females. *Journal of Adolescent Health Care, 6,* 445–447.

Netting, N. (1992). Sexuality in youth culture: Identity and change. *Adolescence, 27,* 961–976.

Newcomer, S., & Udry, J. (1985). Parent-child communication and adolescent sexual behavior. *Family Planning Perspectives, 17,* 169–174.

Norris, A., & Ford, K. (1994). Condom beliefs in urban, low income, African American and Hispanic Youth. *Health Education Quarterly, 21,* 39–53.

Polit-O'Hara, D., & Kahn, J. (1985). Communication and contraceptive practices in adolescent couples. *Adolescence, 20,* 33–43.

Resnick, M., & Blum, R. (1985). Developmental and personalogical correlates of adolescent sexual behavior and outcome. *International Journal of Adolescent Medicine and Health, 1,* 293–313.

Reschovsky, J., & Gerner, J. (1991). Contraceptive choice among teenagers: A multivariate analysis. *Lifestyles: Family and Economic Issues, 12,* 171–194.

Rickert, V. I., Jay, M. S., Gottlieb, A., & Bridges, C. (1989). Adolescents and AIDS. Females' attitudes and behaviors toward condom purchase and use. *Journal of Adolescent Health Care, 10*(4), 313–316.

Scher, P., Emans, S., & Grace, E. (1982). Factors associated with compliance to oral contraceptive use in an adolescent population. *Journal of Adolescent Health Care, 3,* 120–123.

Scott, C., Shifman, L., Orr, L., Owen, R., & Fawcett, N. (1988). Hispanic and black American adolescents' beliefs related to sexuality and contraception. *Adolescence, 23,* 667–688.

SmithBattle, L. (1995). Teenage mothers' narrative of self: An examination of risking the future. *Advances in Nursing Science, 17*(4), 22–36.

Sorenson, R. (1973). *Adolescent sexuality in contemporary America.* New York: World Publishing.

Tanner, J. (1971). Sequence, tempo, and individual variation in growth and development of boys and girls aged 12 to 16. In R. Muuss (Ed.), *Adolescent behavior and society: A book of readings* (pp. 36–52). New York: Random House.

Wadhera, S., & Silins, J. (1990). Teenage pregnancy in Canada, 1975–1987. *Family Planning Perspectives, 22,* 27–30.

Weisman, C., Plichta, S., Nathanson, C., Ensminger, M., & Robinson, J. (1991). Consistency of condom use for disease prevention among adolescent users of oral contraceptives. *Family Planning Perspectives, 23,* 71–74.

White, J. (1987). Influence of parents, peers, and problem-solving on contraceptive use. *Pediatric Nursing, 13,* 317–321.

Whitley, B., & Schofield, J. (1985, 1986). A meta-analysis of research on adolescent contraceptive use. *Population and Environment, 8,* 173–203.

Williams, L., & Pratt, W. (1990). Wanted and unwanted childbearing in the United States: 1973–1988. *Advance data from vital and health statistics* (No. 189). Hyattsville, MD: National Center for Health Statistics.

Winter, L. (1988). The role of sexual self-concept in the use of contraceptives. *Family Planning Perspectives, 20,* 123–127.

Zabin, L., & Clark, S. (1981). Why they delay: A study of teenage family planning clinic patients. *Family Planning Perspectives, 13,* 205–217.

Zabin, L., Stark, H., & Emerson, M. (1991). Reasons for delay in contraceptive clinic utilization. *Journal of Adolescent Health, 12,* 225–232.

Zelnik, M. (1983). Sexual activity among adolescents: Perspectives of a decade. In E. McAnarney (Ed.), *Premature Adolescent Pregnancy and Parenthood* (pp. 21–33). New York: Grune & Stratton.

Zelnik, M., Koenig, M., & Kim, I. (1984). Sources of prescription contraceptives and subsequent pregnancy among young women. *Family Planning Perspectives, 16,* 6–13.

CHAPTER SEVEN

The Contraceptive Needs of Midlife Women

Monica E. Jarrett and Dona J. Lethbridge

Pregnancy is a possibility for approximately 26% of U.S. women between ages 40 and 44 (Fortney, 1987). The latest U.S. statistics, collected in 1988 as part of the National Survey of Family Growth (N.S.F.G.) suggest that of those women using any method of contraception, approximately 48% of women between 35 and 44 have had a tubal sterilization and 21% have partners who have undergone vasectomy (Mosher & Pratt, 1990). Included in female sterilization are the almost 22% who have had a hysterectomy. In addition, 3% are menopausal. Close to 9% of women this age are not heterosexually active, and another 1% are pregnant or postpartum. No U.S. statistics are available for women aged 45 and older. However, statistics collected in Canada in 1984 provide some information about women aged 45 to 49 (Balakrishnan, Krotki, & Lapierre-Adamcyk, 1985). In Canada, 18.5% of women aged 45 to 49 are considered capable of becoming pregnant. These statistics must be compared cautiously with U.S. figures, however, since more women in Canada have undergone sterilization—38% versus 25% for all age groups.

Between the ages of 40 and 50, most women undergo a physiological transition from fertile menstrual cycles to an anovulatory state (Luoto, Kaprio, & Uutela, 1994; Van Keep, Brand, & Lehert, 1979). This transition from fertile to anovulatory menstrual cycles is rife with uncertainty because the pattern of change is typified by years of variable menstrual cycle length and inconsistent fertility. Not only do previously successful strategies for assessing times of fertility become unreliable, but contraceptive methods become increasingly contraindicated, both medically and physiologically.

Contraceptive practices should be reassessed for all women entering midlife who have not been contraceptively sterilized and are still at risk for pregnancy. Moreover, health care providers should educate women about the physiological and functional changes that are a normal part of midlife. Many women in their 40s have completed childbearing and do not plan additional pregnancies. In fact, more than 50% of pregnancies conceived after the age of 40 are terminated through induced abortion (Henshaw, 1987). Yet, despite these realities, procedures for contraceptive use during midlife are less clear and more difficult, and contraceptive choices are more limited than previously. This might explain why greater than 12% of women between the ages of 40 and 44 who are still at risk for pregnancy and sexually active use no method of birth control at all during those years (Fortney, 1987). Women wanting to prevent pregnancy during midlife may need help in choosing a new contraceptive technique that is satisfactory to them and in using it effectively until it is no longer necessary.

There is evidence that fertility wanes during the 40s. When birth rates of large samples of women in historically noncontraceptive-using populations were examined, the results depicted a sharp decrease in births, starting at age 40 (Leridon, 1979; Meneken, Trussell, & Larsen, 1986). A similar trend can still be seen in the U.S. Census statistics. In 1985 there were 4 live births per 1,000 women aged 40 to 44, and 0.2 live births per 1,000 women aged 45 to 49. These statistics represent an 83% and 99% decrease, respectively, from the rate of births found in women 35 to 39 years of age. Contraceptive practices may somewhat influence this decrease in rate of births, but not the overall drop in the curve.

The reason for this rapid decrease in fertility appears to be a change in the hypothalamic-pituitary-ovarian system and uterine integrity. The most obvious sign of this is a change in menstrual cycle length. Treloar et al. (1967) examined the menstrual cycle lengths of women throughout their menstruating years and found that a period of increased variability appears to precede the final cessation of menstruation. This phase has been called the perimenopausal or transition phase. This phase typically begins in the woman's 40s and lasts a mean of six years, although it can last from as short as 1 year to as long as 10 years (Treloar, 1982). During this period, menstrual cycles usually vary from fewer than 26 days to greater than 32 days. Prolonged cycles are not uncommon. Wallace et al. (1979) reported that until a cycle has lasted 210 days in a 45- to 49-year-old women, there is less than a 50% chance that she has actually reached menopause. Kaufert et al. (1987) reported as many as 81 different combination patterns (e.g., regular to irregular to regular cycle lengths) in 324 women who were followed over 3 years.

These wide swings in cycle lengths can be deceptive, especially the prolonged cycles. Treloar noted that false alarms for menopause occurred 40% of the time in a sample of 303 women whose cycles would become variable for a short period and then revert to a more stable ovulatory pattern. Metcalf (1979) found that in a sample of 139 women 40- to 50-years-old, cycles of 21 to 35 days showed pregnanediol changes consistent with ovulation, irrespective of age. Although prolonged cycles were generally anovulatory, this was not always the case. Cycles shorter than 21 days were usually ovulatory.

The feedback mechanisms that regulate the hypothalamic-pituitary-ovarian hormones appear to be altering during the transition phase. Studies of women with regular cycles from age 20 to 50 years show gradual increases in follicle stimulating hormones (FSH) with age (Reyes, Winter, & Faiman, 1977; Sherman & Korenman, 1975; Sherman, West, & Korenman, 1976; Lenton et al., 1988). Luteinizing hormone (LH) levels in these same subjects appear to remain unchanged when assessed by age alone. Notable FSH levels only appear to rise significantly in menstruating women five to 6 years before menopause. When assessed relative to an individual woman's menopause, LH levels rise significantly three to 4 years before menopause. The variability from woman to woman and cycle to cycle makes it difficult to determine an absolute level at which it can be said safely that a woman is no longer fertile. As a rule of thumb, current research suggests that a woman with FSH levels at or above 8 I.U. is probably 6 years or fewer from menopause. LH levels are probably not helpful in making that determination. Prolonged cycles are often associated with elevated FSH and LH levels comparable to those found during menopause.

Midfollicular and midluteal levels of estrogens and midluteal progesterone levels have been reported to be lower than levels in younger women, although these findings are not always consistent. This may be because some cycles have adequate follicular stimulation and maturation, while in others the follicles do not fully ripen and therefore produce less developed corpus lutea.

In the past, the cause of these hormonal changes was hypothesized to be due to a depleting supply and eventual absence of primordial follicles. Costoff and Mahesh (1975) have shown that primordial follicles are still present in postmenopausal women. However, the differentiating follicles appear to be in various states of atresia, thus suggesting that the ovarian follicles are no longer sensitive to gonadotropin stimulation.

Decreased levels of inhibin, a hormone produced by the granulosa cells, have also been implicated in this process, since inhibin is believed to have a suppressive effect on FSH secretion (Sheth & Moodbidri, 1986).

Uterine integrity may also contribute to the decrease in natural fertility found after 40 years of age. Stein (1985) suggests that the uterus loses its ability to support an embryo, either after implantation or at a later developmental stage. There is a dramatic rise in the number of spontaneous abortions (with normal fetal chromosomal patterns) for women, starting in their late 30s.

BELIEFS AND FEELINGS ABOUT FERTILITY

It has been suggested that perimenopausal women do not regret the loss of fertility accompanying menopause (Neugarten et al., 1963; Perlmutter & Bart, 1982). However, these studies have not focused on those women for whom pregnancy is still a possibility, those who have not undergone tubal sterilization, hysterectomy, or whose partner has not undergone vasectomy.

Midlife women who have not been sterilized may have been reluctant to become infertile. There has been, for instance, a striking increase in the number of births for women 35 to 44, from 1,991,000 in 1982 to 2,690,000 in 1988 (Williams & Pratt, 1990). In a qualitative study of 25 potentially fertile midlife women, the women generally considered themselves fertile because they were still having menstrual periods, but acknowledged they did not know for sure (Jarrett & Lethbridge, 1994). In addition to their periods, they used other guides such as their history of having gotten pregnant easily or their mothers' and other relatives' experiences of having pregnancies late in life. Some had more direct evidence of fertility, such as having had a recent pregnancy. For women still wanting to become pregnant, some fertility was assumed, though women recognized that they were probably less fertile than when younger.

On the other hand, even if women are theoretically at risk for pregnancy, they may believe they can no longer conceive and forgo contraceptive use. Luker (1975) has suggested that a woman estimates the probability of becoming pregnant during any single episode of intercourse, and that the longer a woman engages in unprotected intercourse without pregnancy occurring, the more likely she is to continue. Thus, if a woman in midlife has been having unprotected intercourse without becoming pregnant over several cycles, she may mistakenly assume she has become infertile and then become pregnant during a fertile cycle.

CONTRACEPTIVE CHOICES

It is generally recommended that women in their midyears continue to use contraception for 2 years after the cessation of menses if it occurs before age 49, and for 1 year if it occurs after age 50. However, women who are actively using contraception are somewhat limited in the choices available to them.

Generally, birth control pills have been contraindicated in this age group, since the risk of emboli-related myocardial infarction and stroke, as well as hypertension, increases with age. Hormonal replacement therapy, frequently used in postmenopausal women, is generally based on natural estrogens (i.e., conjugated equine estrogens, estradiol valerate or micronized estradiol) that have no effect on diastolic blood pressure and do not promote the development of thrombi, especially when administered via nonoral routes (L'Hermite, Van Pachterbeke, & Van Roosendaal, 1988; Upton, 1987). However, natural estrogens result in poorly controlled menstrual cycles in premenopausal women. Progesterone, particularly androgenic nortestosterone-derived progesterones such as norgestrel and norethisterone, has been related to an increased risk of arterial disease and been found to raise the level of low-density and decrease the level of high-density lipoprotein cholesterol (L'Hermite, Van Pachterbeke, & Van Roosendaal, 1988; W.H.O. Task Force on Oral Contraceptives, 1988). The nonandrogenic progesterones—cyproterone acetate and dydrogesterone—have been shown to not affect changes in cholesterol levels, but to raise levels of serum triglycerides.

Studies in the past linking estrogen formulations with thromboembolitic deaths were performed with higher doses of estrogen than those generally used today, and at a time when there were fewer contraindications in place for oral contraceptive use (Mishell, 1988). More than 75% of oral contraceptive users now take formulations with less than 50 μg of estrogen. A study from 1977 to 1982 of 65,000 oral contraceptive users found no greater incidence of myocardial infarction or cerebrovascular accident among oral contraceptive users who were screened for pre-existing conditions that could predispose them to arterial or venous thrombosis. Women at risk, however, because of pre-exisiting conditions must be properly screened (Bachmann, 1994; Boulanger, Condry, & Devoldere, 1994).

In addition to preventing a midlife pregnancy, the use of birth control pills by midlife women has the benefits of re-establishing a regular menstrual pattern, preventing menopausal symptoms, and retarding osteoporosis. Thus the Fertility and Maternal Health Drugs Advisory

Committee of the FDA suggested that birth control pills with low doses of estrogen may be used for midlife women who do not smoke and are not obese, hypertensive, diabetic, lipidemic, or who have a previous history of thrombosis, heart disease, or pregnancy-induced hypertension.

The N.S.F.G. study done in 1988 found that 2.1% of women 35 to 44 years old who used a reversible form of contraception were using the IUD. For some years, because of media coverage of the risks of IUDs and fear of lawsuits, IUDs had been taken off the American market. However, now the Progestasert IUD, a hormonal IUD with an effective lifetime of 1 year, and a new Copper T IUD are now available. The IUD may be especially appropriate for midlife women, since the fear of pelvic inflammatory disease (PID) with resulting loss of fertility may be less of an issue for women of this age group. The risk of PID is also much lower for women in stable, monogamous relationships (Grimes, 1987). However, problems with menorrhagia or fibroids, or previous cervical surgery would contraindicate its use (Bowen-Simpkins, 1984; Newton, 1988). It is also recommended that the IUD be removed if menopause is imminent, since there is a risk of it imbedding into the uterine wall (Newton, 1988).

The predominant reversible contraceptives used by women aged 35 to 44 who have not, nor has their partner been, sterilized, are barrier methods (Mosher & Pratt, 1990). Thirty-six percent use condoms and 19% use diaphragms or cervical caps. Barrier methods are innately difficult for many women since they must be used during every episode of sexual intercourse. However, the use of contraceptive jelly with a diaphragm or contraceptive foam may be advantageous to midlife women for alleviating the vaginal dryness that perimenopausal women may intermittently suffer because of the periodic decreases in estrogen. The diaphragm may be difficult for some women in their midyears to use if they suffer from pelvic muscular relaxation. The Prentif-Rim cervical cap, approved for use by the FDA since 1988, may be appropriate for midlife women, but retention rates due to difficulty of use, and the availability of only four sizes limit its availability (Powell et al., 1986; Richwald et al., 1989). The condom may present problems for middle-aged partners as penile sensitivity decreases.

Some women have reported using barrier methods in conjunction with the rhythm method, natural family planning, or fertility awareness, thus employing a contraceptive method only when they believe they are in the fertile phase of the menstrual cycle (Lethbridge, 1990; Swanson & Corbin, 1983). The practice is seldom noted in studies of contraceptive use, but may well be prevalent. However, methods of fertility awareness become difficult if not impossible to use during midlife as menstrual cycles increase in variability.

Kippley and Kippley (1979) suggest that natural family planning using the sympto-thermal method of temperature, mucus, and cervical observations is very difficult during the perimenopausal period if the woman has not mastered the technique earlier. Cervical mucus may occur during an anovulatory cycle corresponding to variations in FSH levels and thus estrogen levels, but it will not be clear that it is an anovulatory cycle until after the fact—when the mucus has disappeared and no ovulatory basal body temperature increase has occurred. Endometrial shedding may occur and be indistinguishable from a menstrual period or ovulatory spotting, confounding cyclic observations.

STRATEGIES FOR INTERVENTION

Contraceptive teaching and counseling during midlife in those women, or those with partners, who have not undergone a sterilization procedure is complex because of the unpredictable physiological status and additional constraints that aging might bring. However, there is some evidence that during midlife because of very apparent physical changes, women may be more aware of health needs and attuned to health promotion behaviors (Hartweg, 1993).

During assessment, contraceptive needs and, as much as possible, women's fertility status should be evaluated. An assessment of menstrual patterns would ideally include the length of cycles for the past 12 months; length and nature of menstrual flow, such as number of tampons or napkins per day, and any changes in cycle length, flow, or onset of spotting; metrorrhagia; or dysmennorhea. Many women do not keep records of or accurately remember past their most recent menstrual cycle (Bean et al., 1979). A woman should be encouraged to make a yearly record, either in the form of a Treloar-type card (see Table 7.1) or on a personal calendar, possibly modified to include menstrual cycle detail (Becker & Sosa, 1992). A computerized calendar has been developed that enables a woman to record menstrual history and fertility symptoms (Taylor, Lugan, & Vazquez-Geffroy, 1995). Although this approach would be appropriate only for certain computer-comfortable women, it has shown to be an efficient and accurate way to collect data.

Sampling blood FSH levels at any single point in time does not adequately define a woman as menopausal, although it might be suggestive

TABLE 7.1. Menstrual Calendar for Recording Menstrual Cycles

Circle each menstrual date or join circled first and last dates. Dot above indicates spotting.

Calendar Year

January																											
1	2	3	4	5	6	7	8	9	10	11	12	13	14	15	16	17	18	19	20	21	22	23	24	25	26	27	28
29	30	31	**February** 1	2	3	4	5	6	7	8	9	10	11	12	13	14	15	16	17	18	19	20	21	22	23	24	25
26	27	28	**March** 1	2	3	4	5	6	7	8	9	10	11	12	13	14	15	16	17	18	19	20	21	22	23	24	25
26	27	28	29	30	31	**April** 1	2	3	4	5	6	7	8	9	10	11	12	13	14	15	16	17	18	19	20	21	22
23	24	25	26	27	28	29	30	**May** 1	2	3	4	5	6	7	8	9	10	11	12	13	14	15	16	17	18	19	20
21	22	23	24	25	26	27	28	29	30	31	**June** 1	2	3	4	5	6	7	8	9	10	11	12	13	14	15	16	17
18	19	20	21	22	23	24	25	26	27	28	29	30	**July** 1	2	3	4	5	6	7	8	9	10	11	12	13	14	15
16	17	18	19	20	21	22	23	24	25	26	27	28	29	30	31	**August** 1	2	3	4	5	6	7	8	9	10	11	12
13	14	15	16	17	18	19	20	21	22	23	24	25	26	27	28	29	30	31	**September** 1	2	3	4	5	6	7	8	9
10	11	12	13	14	15	16	17	18	19	20	21	22	23	24	25	26	27	28	29	30	**October** 1	2	3	4	5	6	7
8	9	10	11	12	13	14	15	16	17	18	19	20	21	22	23	24	25	26	27	28	29	30	31	**November** 1	2	3	4
5	6	7	8	9	10	11	12	13	14	15	16	17	18	19	20	21	22	23	24	25	26	27	28	29	30	**December** 1	2
3	4	5	6	7	8	9	10	11	12	13	14	15	16	17	18	19	20	21	22	23	24	25	26	27	28	29	30
31	**January** 1	2	3	4	5	6	7	8	9	10	11	12	13	14	15	16	17	18	19	20	21	22	23	24	25	26	27

Calendar adapted from Treloar (1967) by Tremin Trust Program on Women's Health, University of Utah, College of Nursing, Salt Lake City.

104

of approaching menopause if the level is 8 IU or greater. Blood levels of LH are not useful, but an LH to FSH ratio of less than one suggests that menopause is probably less than 6 years away (Bachmann, 1994). Other factors enabling the prediction of the onset of menopause are given in Table 7.2.

It is important that women's knowledge about their own fertility be assessed. Once menstrual cycles have started to increase in length, women may assume they have become menopausal and are no longer fertile. Even without noticeable menstrual changes, they may also assume this once they have passed the age of 40. On the other hand, sporadically increased cycle lengths may lead women to think they are pregnant, which may be anxiety producing in many cases. It is important that women be aware not only of the changes in menstrual patterns they

TABLE 7.2. Correlates of Early or Late Menopause Related to Information Gathered During the History

Age at menopause for women in general
Median age 49–50 years

Family history
No correlation between mother's and daughter's age at menopause
Personal characteristics
Nutritional state of mother at time of the pregnancy may be important; poor prenatal nutrition seems to lead to daughter's earlier menopause.
Nutritional state of women, for example, lean and small women tend to experience menopause earlier, heavy and short women later
Low economic status—earlier menopause
Contraceptive practice—many years of oral contraceptive use may lead to slightly later onset of menopause
Smoking—more than 15 cigarettes a day correlates with earlier menopause
Blindness—later onset of menopause

Pathology
Precocious menopause may occur with the following:
Genetic factors: Turner's syndrome (XO) or XX/XO mosaicism; trisomies (XXX), chromosomes 18 and 21; familial inherited chromosome defect that is rare
Autoimmune disease: may occur in Addison's disease, hypoparathyroidism, and Hashimoto's thyroiditis; chronic yeast infections (Candida sp.)
Cytotoxic drugs
Ionizing radiation

Adapted from Gorden, R. G.: *Biology of menopause: The causes and consequences of ovarian aging,* New York, Academic Press, 1985.

may expect or may be experiencing, but also the implications of these changes for their fertility.

It is important to assess women's plans and feelings about future pregnancies. Positive feelings about the waning or loss of fertility should not be assumed. Women who are still at risk for pregnancy during midlife are those who have decided not to undergo tubal sterilization. Though there may be reasons such as reluctance to undergo surgery or satisfaction with a current contraceptive choice, some women may not have made a definitive decision about their fertility. Some women's new awareness of the means of extending fertility may also need to be addressed, including the many issues, including social, financial, and ethical, that might impact such a course (Chalmers, 1994; Frank, Bianchi, & Campana, 1994). Ambivalent feelings about future pregnancies or the loss of fertility may place women at risk for abandoning the use of contraceptives and having an unplanned and ill-timed conception.

CONCLUSION

For women in midlife, contraceptive choices are limited. Women may be in the position of needing to change to a less preferable method, making contraceptive use more difficult because women may also realize that they may no longer be fertile. Some may cope with this difficulty by using no contraception in the hope that it is not needed. It is essential, in this situation, that women be helped to select contraceptive techniques that are as satisfactory as possible. This necessitates consideration of a woman's physiological status as well as her personal preferences. The health care practitioner should also discuss with women whether or not they would undergo an abortion if pregnancy occurred. If abortion is not an option, more reliable contraception is called for.

REFERENCES

Bachmann, G. A. (1994). The change before 'the change.' Strategies for the transition to the menopause. *Post-graduate Medicine, 95*(4), 113–115, 119–121, 124.

Balakrishnan, T. R., Krotki, K., & Lapierre-Adamcyk, E. (1985). Contraceptive use in Canada, 1984, *Family Planning Perspectives, 17,* 209–215.

Bean, J. A., Leeper, J. D., Wallace, R. B., Sherman, B. M., & Jaggar, H. (1979). Variations in the reporting of menstrual histories. *American Journal of Epidemiology, 109*(2), 181–185.

Becker, S., & Sosa, D. (1992). An experiment using a month-by-month calendar in a family planning survey in Costa Rica. *Studies in Family Planning, 23,* 386–391.

Boulanger, J. C., Gondry, J., & Devoldere, K. (1994). A qual age faut-il arreter la contraception orale? [At what age should oral contraception be stopped?] *Review of French Gynecologie-Obstetrique, 89*(7–9), 409–413.

Bowen-Simkins, P. (1984). Contraception for the older woman. *British Journal of Obstetrics and Gynecology, 91,* 513–515.

Chalmers, C. (1994). Fertility and the menopause. *British Journal of Nursing, 3*(9), 450–4453.

Costoff, A., & Mahesh, V. (1975). Primordial follicles with normal oocytes in the ovaries of postmenopausal women. *American Geriatrics Society, 23,* 193–196.

Fortney, J. A. (1987). Contraception for American women 40 and over. *Family Planning Perspectives, 19,* 32–34.

Frank, O., Bianchi, P. G., & Campana, A. (1994). The end of fertility, age, fecundity and fecundability in women. *Journal of Biosocial Science, 26*(3), 349–368.

Grimes, D. (1987). Intrauterine devices and pelvic inflammatory diseases: Recent developments. *Contraception, 36,* 97–109.

Hartweg, D. L. (1993). Self-care actions of healthy middle-aged women to promote well-being. *Nursing Research, 42,* 221–227.

Henshaw, S. K. (1987). Characteristics of U.S. women having abortions, 1982–1983. *Family Planning Perspectives, 19,* 5–9.

Jarrett, M. E., & Lethbridge, D. J. (1994). Looking forward, looking back: Women's experience with waning fertility during mid-life. *Qualitative Health Research, 4,* 370–384.

Kaufert, P., Gilbert, G., & Tate, R. (1987). Defining menopausal status: The impact of longitudinal data. *Maturitas, 9,* 217–226.

Kippley, J., & Kippley, S. (1979). *The art of natural family planning.* Cincinnati: The Couple to Couple League.

L'Hermite, M., Van Pachterbeke, C., & Van Roosendaal, E. (1988). From oral contraception to hormone replacement therapy: Towards a continuum? *Maturitas (Suppl.), 1,* 155–165.

Leridon, H. (1979). Patterns of fertility at later ages of reproduction. *Journal of Biosocial Science, (Suppl.), 6,* 59–74.

Lethbridge, D. J. (1990). The contraceptive use of women of upper socioeconomic status. *Health Care for Women International, 11,* 305–318.

Luker, K. (1975). *Taking chances: Abortion and the decision not to contracept.* Berkeley, CA: University of California Press.

Luoto, R., Kaprio, J., & Uutela, A. (1994). Age at natural menopause and sociodemographic status in Finland. *American Journal of Epidemiology, 139*(1), 64–76.

Meneken, J., Trussell, J., & Larsen, U. (1986). Age and infertility. *Science, 233,* 1389–1394.

Metcalfe, M. (1979). Incidence of ovulatory cycles in women approaching the menopause. *Journal of Biosocial Science, 11,* 39–48.

Mosher, W. D., & Pratt, W. F. (1990). Contraceptive use in the United States, 1973—1988. *Advance data from vital and health statistics; No. 182.* Hyattsville, MD: National Center for Health Statistics.

Mishell, D. R. (1988). Use of oral contraceptives in women of older reproductive age. *American Journal of Obstetrics and Gynecology, 142,* 1652–1657.

Neugarten, B. L., Wood, V. J., Kraines, R. J., & Loomis, B. (1963). Women's attitudes toward the menopause. *Vita Humana, 6,* 140–151.

Newton, J. (1988). Contraception for the woman aged 35 years and over. *Maturitas (Suppl.), 1,* 89–98.

Perlmutter, E., & Bart, P. B. (1982). Changing views of "The change": A critical review and suggestions for an attributional approach. In A. M. Voda, M. Dinnerstein, & S. R. O'Donnell (Eds.), *Changing perspectives on menopause* (pp. 257–266). Austin, TX: University of Texas Press.

Powell, M. G., Mears, B. J., Deber, R. B., & Ferguson, D. (1986). Contraception with the cervical cap: Effectiveness, safety, continuity of use, and user satisfaction. *Contraception, 33,* 215–232.

Reyes, F. I., Winter, J. S., & Faiman, C. (1977). I. A cross-sectional study of serum follicle-stimulating hormone, luteinizing hormone, prolactin, estradiol, and progesterone levels. *American Journal of Obstetrics and Gynecology, 129,* 557–564.

Richwald, G. A., Greenland, S., Gerber, M. M., Potik, R., Kersey, A., & Comas, M. A. (1989). Effectiveness of the cavity rim cervical cap: Results of a large clinical study. *Obstetrics and Gynecology, 74,* 143–148.

Sherman, B. M., & Korenman, S. G. (1975). Hormonal characteristics of the human menstrual cycle throughout reproductive life. *Journal of Clinical Investigation, 55,* 699–706.

Sherman, B. M., West, J. H., & Korenman, S. G. (1976). The menopausal transition: Analysis of LH, FSH, Estradiol, and Progesterone concentrations during menstrual cycles of older women. *Journal of Clinical Endocrinology and Metabolism, 42,* 629–636.

Sheth, A. R., & Moodbidri, S. B. (1986). Potential application of inhibin in male and female contraception. *Advances in Contraception, 2,* 131–139.

Stein, Z. A. (1985). Review and commentary. A woman's age: Childbearing and childrearing. *American Journal of Epidemiology, 121,* 327–342.

Swanson, J. M., & Corbin, J. (1983). The contraceptive context: A model for increasing nursing's involvement in family health. *Maternal-Child Nursing Journal, 12,* 169–183.

Taylor, B., Lujan, P., & Vazquez-Geffrey, M. (1995). An event recorder for infant feeding research. *Computer Methods and Programs in Biomedicine, 47*(3), 267–274.

Treloar, A. E., Boynton, R. D., Behn, B. G., & Brown, B. W. (1967). Variation of the human menstrual cycle through reproductive life. *International Journal of Fertility, 12,* 77–126.

Treloar, A. (1982). Predicting the close of menstrual life. In A. M. Voda, M. Dinnerstein, & S. R. O'Donnell (Eds.), *Changing perspectives on menopause.* Austin, TX: University of Texas Press, 77–126.

Upton, G. V. (1987). Contraception for the perimenopausal patient. *Obstetric and Gynecologic Clinics of North America, 14*(1), 207–227.

Van Keep, P. A., Brand, P. C., & Lehert, P. L. (1979). Factors affecting the age at menopause. *Journal of Biosocial Science, (Suppl.), 6,* 37–55.

Wallace, R. B., Sherman, B. M., Bean, J. A., Treloar, A. E., Schlabaugh, L. (1979). Probability of menopause with increasing duration of amenorrhea in middle-aged women. *American Journal of Obstetrics and Gynecology, 135,* 1021–1024.

W.H.O. Task Force on Oral Contraceptives. (1988). A multicentre comparative study of serum lipids and lipoproteins in four groups of combined contraceptive users and a control group of IUD users. *Contraception, 38,* 605–629.

Williams, L. B., & Pratt, W. F. (1990). Wanted and unwanted childbearing in the United States: 1973–1988. *Advance Data from Vital and Health Statistics of the National Center for Health Statistics, no. 189.* Hyattsville, MD: National Center for Health Statistics.

The Choice of Contraceptive Methods Available

The chapters in this part cover and list the contraceptive methods currently available. The first chapter includes factors to be considered when examining contraceptive data. The remaining chapters each discuss a category of methods. Included in each is the physiological effect including mechanism of action, side effects, and contraindications, efficacy rates, factors that impact their correct and consistent use, and women's and men's experience with using the method.

Factors to Consider When Examining Contraceptive Data

Dona J. Lethbridge and Kathleen M. Hanna

The plain and simple purpose of contraception is to prevent unwanted pregnancies. Unwanted pregnancies are traumatic for any woman or couple. It is important to define, however, the term "unwanted" and be sure that it is distinguished from "unplanned" or "unintended."

It is also important to distinguish pregnancies that are perceived as unwanted by the women carrying them from those perceived as undesirable by society. A pregnancy considered socially undesirable or unwanted, may, in fact, be wanted by the individual woman. For instance, of those births to never-married women aged 15 to 19 years, 76.8% were reported as wanted (though unplanned or mistimed) at conception (Williams & Pratt, 1990). Yet, many people would consider these conceptions as undesirable, and unwanted by the larger society. Over 837,000 teenage pregnancies were estimated for the year 1988, 23,000 to those aged 14 and younger (Trussell & Kost, 1987). Of these pregnancies, only 16% are intended, that is, purposefully conceived.

Feelings about how much a pregnancy is wanted may change throughout the course of the pregnancy. In a classic theoretical paper, Pohlman (1965) discussed the concept of unwanted pregnancy. At conception, a pregnancy might have been unplanned and undesired but later, as the pregnancy progressed, accepted and wanted. The first trimester of pregnancy may be a time of ambivalence when, regardless of whether the conception was planned and wanted, feelings of happiness are accompanied by feelings of regret and even panic.

To prevent unwanted pregnancies, providers need to be knowledge-able about contraceptive methods and their effectiveness. Family planning practitioners have been shown to have an inclination to over-estimate the efficacy of methods they prefer, such as hormonal techniques, and to under-estimate the efficacy of methods they disfa-vor, such as barrier methods (Trussell, Faden, & Hatcher, 1976). It is incumbent on providers to be aware that all methods have a surprising-ly high effectiveness rate if they are used correctly and consistently. It is more important that a method be one women and men can use, even if its effectiveness rate is a little lower than other methods. Providers must be able to knowledgeably examine and critique contraceptive data as it is gathered, especially in relation to user effectiveness rates.

A variety of contraceptive methods are used in the United States (see Table 8.1). The predominant methods are reported by the National Survey of Family Growth (N.S.F.G.), with the most recent findings from the 1988 study (Mosher & Pratt, 1990). In that survey, 8,460 women, randomly sampled, were interviewed regarding their contraceptive use. In cases where use of more than one method is reported, the most effective method is attributed to the woman and tabulated. Thus, sta-tistics are probably more accurate for hormonal contraceptives or the IUD, both of which tend to be used solely, but much less representa-tive of methods considered ineffective such as fertility awareness, withdrawal, or douching, when they are used on subsequent days alternating with other more effective methods.

The N.S.F.G. reports that of women who use no contraception even though they are not trying to become pregnant, 40% will conceive within 1 year. This is lower than the generally reported and accepted 80 to 85% (Trussell & Kost, 1987). The N.S.F.G., however, does not collect data on reasons for nonuse, such as a history of infertility or "success-fully avoiding pregnancy while not using birth control."

Statistics on unwanted pregnancies are also skewed, in that data are reported as unwanted conceptions at the time of pregnancy for births occurring within the last 5 years. Unwanted pregnancies that result in abortions are not included in the analysis.

The most recent N.S.F.G. was conducted between January and October, 1995, and it is expected that initial findings probably will be available in early 1997 (Mosher & Bachrach, 1996). In that survey, some changes were made: More explanatory measures were added, to help elucidate relationships between variables. Personal history data have been added, including marriages, divorces, and sexual partner-ships as well as questions on attitudes toward marriage and childbear-ing. Because the survey is now longer, a $20.00 incentive has been

TABLE 8.1.   Predominant Contraceptive Methods Used by Women 15 to 44 in the United States, 1988, from the National Survey of Family Growth (%)

Method	Hispanic	Non-Hispanic White	Non-Hispanic African American
Female sterilization	32	26	38
Male sterilization	4	14	1
Pill	33	30	38
IUD	5	2	3
Diaphragm	2	7	2
Condom	14	15	10

Source: Mosher & Pratt (1990).

added for participation. Computer-assisted interviewing has also been added to reduce interviewer error. This has also enabled the addition of more personal questions such as histories of induced abortions and other sensitive topics. In the latest survey, women were able to answer sensitive questions themselves, listening to the questions on audio headphones and answering directly into the computer. Thus, when the new N.S.F.G. data are available, the information will be more comprehensive and qualitatively improved.

Another issue related to the reporting of contraceptive data relates to the failure of contraceptive methods. Three types of contraceptive failure rates are reported. Extended-use failure rates include all pregnancies and exposures that occur while the method is being used or after the method has been discontinued for any reason other than intent to conceive. Actual use failure rates include failures and exposure that occur while the method is being used under both correct conditions and imperfectly in some way. These are also referred to as user failure rates. Method failure rates include only conceptions and exposures occurring during correct and consistent use. It is informative to compare differences between user failures and method failures, since this gives an estimate of difficulty of use (see Table 8.2).

Contraceptive effectiveness may be defined as "the proportional reduction in fecundability (the monthly probability of conception)" resulting from the use of a method (Trussell et al., 1990, p. 558). In the literature, two methods of measuring contraceptive effectiveness are used: the Pearl index and life table techniques.

The Pearl index is the number of failures of a method per 100 woman-years of exposure. The numerator is the number of unintended pregnancies; the denominator is the total months or cycles of exposure

**TABLE 8.2.   An Estimate of Contraceptive Difficulty, Based on Lowest
Expected and Typical Percentages of Accidental Pregnancy
During the First Year of Use of a Method**

Method	Lowest expected (%) or perfect use	Typical (%)
Chance	85	85
Spermicides	6	21
Fertility awareness		20
Calendar	9	
Ovulation method	3	
Symptothermal	2	
Postovulation	1	
Withdrawal	4	19
Cervical cap		36
Parous women	26	18
Nulliparous women	9	
Diaphragm	6	18
Condom		
Male	3	12
Female (Reality)	5	21
IUD		
Progestasert	1.5	2
Copper T 380A	0.6	0.8
LNg 20	0.1	0.1
Birth control pill		3
Combined	0.1	
Progestogen only	0.5	
Injectable progestogen	0.3	0.3
Implants—Norplant	0.09	0.09
Female sterilization	0.4	0.4
Male sterilization	0.1	0.15

From Hatcher, R. A., Trussell, J., Stewart, F., Stewart, G. K., Kowal, D., Guest, F., Cates, W., & Policar, M. S. *Contraceptive Technology* (16th ed.). New York: Irvington Publishers, Inc., 1994. Reprinted with permission.

until the completion of the study, an unintended pregnancy, or discontinuation of the method. The quotient is multiplied by 1,200 if the denominator consists of months, or if menstrual cycles are used. An inherent problem with the Pearl index is that since calculations are based on varying lengths of time, unintended pregnancy rates may be incomparable. Failure rates of a method decline with use, probably because of learning and that those who do fail with it, drop out early. In comparing failure rates of methods, then, it is important to know the duration of exposure, and they should be the same across methods.

Life table techniques calculate a separate failure rate for each month of use. A cumulative failure rate is constructed showing the proportion of women who fail within any given time. Most frequent in the literature is 12 months. Analyses may be presented as net rates (multiple-decrement life tables) or gross rates (single-decrement life tables). Net rates include failures that have occurred for a variety of reasons—accidental pregnancy, early discontinuation, loss to follow-up. Therefore, net rates cannot be used to compare methods, since each differs in factors that might lead to early discontinuation or pregnancy. Gross rates eliminate any woman who leaves the study for any reason other than accidental pregnancy. Thus, they allow comparison across methods.

Studies can be confounded by women participants' previous contraceptive use. For instance, subfecundity is expected after discontinuing birth control pills, and is even more pronounced after discontinuing injectable hormonal contraception. Previous experience with a method also may affect outcome—the first month of observation in a study may not be the first month of use. Participants may vary in experience. Some methods involve training periods, such as fertility awareness. In some reports of effectiveness, rates are calculated on those who have completed a training period. Failures are probably more likely to occur during the training period, and would then be omitted. If the intent is to compare methods, training time failure rates should also be included, since that period is not omitted from other method studies. Studies of other methods such as withdrawal would benefit from distinction between experienced and inexperienced users. When this was one of the only methods of contraception available and used by many, it might well have been a relatively effective method when couples became experienced. Presently, this method is frequently used by those having their first sexual experiences, with no other contraceptive method perceived to be available. When used by inexperienced and young users, the method is probably very difficult to use effectively.

Another factor to be taken into account when evaluating efficacy rates is the type of user to which they are being applied. Contraceptive failures are generally more likely to occur early in their use. Motivation or intent to avoid pregnancy is another variable. In a study of upper socioeconomic status, professional women, fewer unplanned pregnancies occurred when compared to national norms, and they were more likely to use methods considered less effective, such as withdrawal or fertility awareness, and use them successfully (Lethbridge, 1990).

Similarly, in studies of women in other countries, those women with educational and occupational success have lower fertility rates, in spite of less effective contraception such as barrier methods.

REFERENCES

Hatcher, R. A., Trussell, J., Stewart, F., Stewart, G. K., Kowed, D., Guest, F., Coates, W., & Policer, M. (1996). *Contraceptive technology 1994–1996.* New York: Irvington Press.
Lethbridge, D. J. (1990). Use of contraceptives by women of upper socioeconomic status. *Health Care for Women International, 11,* 305–318.
Mosher, W. D., & Bachrach, C. A. (1996). Understanding U.S. fertility: Continuity and change in the National Survey of Family Growth, 1988–1995. *Family Planning Perspectives, 28*(1), 4–12.
Mosher, W. D., & Pratt, W. F. (1990). Contraceptive use in the United States, 1973–1988. *Advance data from vital and health statistics, No. 182.* Hyattsville, MD: National Center for Health Statistics.
Pohlman, E. (1965). "Unwanted" and "wanted" conceptions: Toward a less ambiguous definition. *Eugenics Quarterly, 12,* 19–27.
Trussell, J., & Kost, K. (1987). Contraceptive failure in the United States: A critical review of the literature. *Studies in Family Planning, 18,* 237–283.
Trussell, J., Faden, R., & Hatcher, R. A. (1976). Efficacy information in contraceptive counseling: those little white lies. *American Journal of Public Health, 66,* 761–767.
Trussell, J., Hatcher, R. A., Cates, Jr., W., Stewart, F. H., & Kost, K. (1990). A guide to interpreting contraceptive efficacy studies. *Obstetrics & Gynecology, 76,* 558–567.
Williams, L. B., & Pratt, W. F. (1990). Wanted and unwanted childbearing in the United States: 1973–1988. *Advance data from vital and health statistics of the national center for health statistics, No. 189.* Hyattsville, MD: National Center for Health Statistics.

C H A P T E R   N I N E

Hormonal Contraceptives

Kathleen M. Hanna

Hormonal contraceptives are safe, effective, and popular. In fact, they are safer than pregnancy, which accounts for more reproductive deaths than does contraception (Grimes, 1994). Hormonal contraceptives are effective when used correctly and consistently (see Table 9.1). Among 15- to 44-year-old women in the United States, oral contraceptives (OCs) are the most popular method when compared with sterilization, intrauterine devices, diaphragms, and condoms (Mosher, 1990).

Hormonal contraceptives are composed of estrogen and/or progestin compounds and may be administered orally, by injections, or via implants (see Table 9.2). OCs may be combined, monophasic, multiphasic, or progestin only. Combined OCs contain both estrogen and progestin and may be of a fixed (monophasic) or variable (multiphasic) dosages. The hormones are taken for 21 days with 7 days between cycles. Some packets have 28 pills—21 with hormonal compounds and 7 blank pills. Progestin-only pills are taken continuously (28 to 42 pills per packet) without any break between cycles. The injectable contraceptive, Depo-Provera, is a progestin compound and is given every 3 months. The implant contraceptive, Norplant, consists of 6 silicone rubber capsules that release progestin at a slow, steady rate (Liskin & Blackburn, 1987).

The main contraceptive mechanism is inhibition of ovulation. Combined OCs have their primary effect on the pituitary. The combined effect of estrogen and progestin inhibits ovulation by suppressing the

TABLE 9.1. Expected Failure Rates for Hormonal Contraceptives During First Year of Use

Oral contraceptives (%)		Injectables (%)		Implants (%)	
Combined	Progestin only	DMPA	NET	Capsules	Rods
0.1	0.5	0.3	0.4	0.04	0.03

Note. Failure rates assume correct and consistent use.
Source: Trussell et al., "Contraceptive Failure in the United States: An Update," Studies in *Family Planning,* 21, no. 1 (Jan/Feb 1990:52).

gonadotropin-producing cells of the pituitary which inhibit the release of gonadotropin-releasing hormones from the hypothalamus (Lobo & Stanczyk, 1994).

The progestin-only contraceptives have their primary effect on the hypothalamus. Progestin decreases the follicle-stimulating hormone level and suppresses the midcycle surge of luteinizing hormones which inhibits ovulation (Darney, 1994; Kaunitz, 1994; Lobo & Stanczyk, 1994). However, ovulation may occur with the progestin-only contraceptives (Darney, 1994; Kaunitz, 1989). The contraceptive mechanism of progestin also involves increasing the thickness of cervical mucus, which inhibits movement of sperm up the reproductive tract and inhibiting endometrial growth for implantation (Darney, 1994; Lobo & Stanczyk, 1994).

Hormonal contraceptive methods are reversible; however, restoration of fertility varies with method. After discontinuation or removal, fertility is restored within an average of 2 months with OCs (Grimes, 1992), 4.5 months with injectables (Kaunitz, 1994), and 1 month with implants (Darney, 1994).

ASSESSMENT

Assessment of health status along with a health history needs to be conducted. The exam should include a pelvic exam with pap smear and measurement of weight and blood pressure (Hatcher et al., 1994). The health history needs to especially focus on the cardiovascular and reproductive systems. Within these systems, there are risks and benefits of using hormonal contraceptives (see Table 9.3). If there are cardiovascular disease (CVD) risks, the health assessment should include a lipid profile and fasting glucose level (Hatcher et al., 1994).

TABLE 9.2.   Examples of Hormonal Contraceptives and Dosages

Contraceptive	Estrogen (in μg)	Progestin (in mg)
Combined monophasics		
Loestrin 1/20	ethinyl estradiol 20	norethindrone acetate 1.0
Norinyl 1/50	mestranol 50	norethindrone 1.0
Ortho 1/50	mestranol 50	norethindrone 1.0
Nordette	ethinyl estradiol 30	levonorgestrel 0.15
Ortho-Cept	ethinyl estradiol 30	desogestrel 0.15
Ortho-Cyclen	ethinyl estradiol 30	norgestimate 0.25
Lo/ovral	ethinyl estradiol 30	norgestrel 0.3
Loestrin 1.5/30	ethinyl estradiol 30	norethindrone acetate 1.5
Ovcon 35	ethinyl estradiol 35	norethindrone 0.4
Brevicon	ethinyl estradiol 35	norethindrone 0.5
Modicom	ethinyl estradiol 35	norethindrone 0.5
Norinyl 1/35	ethinyl estradiol 35	norethindrone 1.0
Ortho 1/35	ethinyl estradiol 35	norethindrone 1.0
Demulen 1/35	ethinyl estradiol 35	ethynodiol diacetate 1.0
Ovcon 50	ethinyl estradiol 50	norethindrone 1.0
Norlestin 1/50	ethinyl estradiol 50	norethindrone acetate 1.0
Ovral	ethinyl estradiol 50	norgestrel 0.5
Demulen 1/50	ethinyl estradiol 50	ethynodiol diacetate 1.0
Combined multiphasic		
Triphasil	ethinyl estradiol 30/40/30	levonorgestrel 0.05/0.075/0.125
Ortho-Tri-Cyclen	ethinyl estradiol 35	norgestimate 0.18/0.215/0.25
Ortho 10/11	ethinyl estradiol 35	norethindrone 0.5/1.0/0.5
Tri-Norinyl	ethinyl estradiol 35	norethindrone 0.5/1.0/0.5
Ortho 7/7/7	ethinyl estradiol 35	norethindrone 0.5/0.75/1.0
Progestin only pills		
Micronor		norethindrone 0.35
Nor-QD		norethindrone 0.35
Ovrette		norgestrel 0.075
Implants		
Norplant		levonorgestrel, 6 capsules @ 36/capsule
Injectables		
Depo-Provera or DMPA		depot medroxyprogesterone acetate 150

Sources: Hatcher et al. (1994); Kaunitz (1994); Liskin & Blackburn (1987); and *Physicians' Desk Reference* (1995).

TABLE 9.3. Potential Health Risks and Benefits of Hormonal Contraceptives

Potential health risks of hormonal contraceptives

Thromboembolism
Pulmonary embolisms
Stroke
Heart disease
Increased cholesterol and trigylcerides
Increased blood pressure
Coagulation and anti-coagulation disorders
Gallbladder disease
Changes in carbohydrate metabolism and diabetes
Liver cancer (inconclusive)
Hepatocellular adenoma (noncancerous liver tumor)
Breast cancer (inconclusive)
Cervical cancer (inconclusive)

Potential noncontraceptive health benefits

Prevention of ectopic pregnancy
Reduction of pelvic inflammatory disease
Decreased menstrual flow
Reduction of iron-deficiency anemia
Less dysmenorrhea
Less premenstrual syndrome
Protection from endometrial cancer
Protection from ovarian cancer
Protection from benign breast disease
Protection from ovarian cysts

Sources: Althaus & Kaeser (1990); Burkman (1994); Darney (1994); Herbst & Berek (1993); Godsland & Crook (1994); Grimes (1992); Kaunitz (1994); Liskin & Blackburn (1987); Mishell (1993); Wharton & Blackburn (1988); and Youngkin (1993).

RISKS AND BENEFITS OF USING HORMONAL CONTRACEPTIVES

Cardiovascular System

There is a risk of cardiovascular disease (CVD) for users of hormonal contraceptives; however, the risk is less with newer compounds. Most of the CVD risks have been documented with older OCs ($\geq$ 50 mcg of estrogen), whereas the risk is minimal with newer low-dose OCs ($\leq$ 35 mcg of estrogen) and progestin-only contraceptives (Darney, 1994; Godsland, Crook, & Wynn, 1992; Grimes, 1992; Samsioe, 1994). Age (> 35 years) is no longer considered a risk for OC use (Stenchever, 1993).

The CVD risks are thromboembolism, heart disease, and stroke (Wharton & Blackburn, 1988). The major risk is thromboembolism, which usually occurs in deep leg veins and sometimes dislodges to become a pulmonary embolism (Wharton & Blackburn, 1988). Thromboembolism is probably the cause of heart disease rather than atherosclerosis as estrogen may provide protection from atherosclerosis (Sullivan & Lobo, 1993).

Many of the risks are associated with CVD risk factors. OCs affect (although minimally) blood pressure (Sullivan & Lobo, 1994), coagulation factors (Samsioe, 1994), and carbohydrate metabolism (Godsland & Crook, 1994). CVD risk increases as high-density lipoproteins (HDL) decreases (< 35 mg/dl), low-density lipoproteins (LDL) increases, and triglycerides increase (> 250 mg/dl) (Godsland, Crook, & Wynn, 1992). Estrogen increases HDL while progestin decreases HDL; however, newer progestin in combination with estrogen does not affect HDL (Godsland & Crook, 1994). HDL and LDL are not changed by implants (Darney, 1994; Shoupe & Mishell, 1989) while the effect of injectables is inconclusive (Kaunitz, 1994). Triglyceride levels are increased in users of combined OCs and may be decreased with implants (Godsland & Crook, 1994). Other risk factors include a family history of heart disease, hypertension, diabetes, smoking, and over 130% of ideal weight (Knopp, LaRosa, & Burkman, 1993).

Reproductive System

Reproductive risks and benefits also exist for users of hormonal contraceptives (see Table 9.3). There is a risk for some cancers (although inconclusive) while there is protection against other cancers. In addition, there are numerous menstrual cycle benefits. There is a lower risk of ectopic pregnancies and ovarian cysts with OCs (Grimes, 1992), an increased risk for ovarian cysts with implants (Darney, 1994), and an increased risk for ectopic pregnancies and ovarian cysts with progestin-only pills (Hatcher et al., 1994).

The association between hormonal contraceptives and sexually transmitted diseases is inconclusive (Cates & Stone, 1992). It has been suggested that the risk of chlamydia is higher since OCs cause cervical tissue to be more vulnerable (Cates & Stone, 1992; Hatcher et al., 1994). In addition, the association between OC use and contraction of human immunodeficiency virus (HIV) is inconclusive (Cates & Stone, 1992; McGregor & Hammill, 1993). However, the risk of contracting HIV is higher among those who have had sexually transmitted diseases such as syphilis and genital herpes as they produce genital ulcers (McGregor & Hammill, 1993).

Hormonal contraceptives provide protection from pelvic inflammatory disease (PID) (Burkman, 1994; Cates & Stone, 1992; Kaunitz, 1994; McGregor & Hammill, 1993). It has been suggested that PID protection is due to progestin effects of: (1) production of thick cervical mucus, which inhibits movement of bacteria to the upper reproductive tract, and (2) decreased menstruation and retrograde flow, which provides a less optimum environment for bacterial growth (Burkman, 1994; Cates & Stone, 1992; McGregor & Hammill, 1993).

Childbearing risks are minimal. Congenital anomalies and prematurity are not risks for infants who are conceived while using or after discontinuing OCs (Liskin & Rutledge, 1984; Liskin & Blackburn, 1987). Combined OCs do inhibit lactation (Wharton & Blackburn, 1988); however, if begun after lactation is established, infant growth and development is not affected (Erwin, 1994). However, OCs are not recommended until after weaning the infant (Physicians' Desk Reference [PDR], 1995).

Other Systems

Hormonal contraceptives impact other systems. Table 9.3 includes the risks and benefits for systems other than cardiovascular and reproductive systems.

STRATEGIES FOR INTERVENTION

DECISION MAKING

Education with counseling may facilitate women's and their partner's contraceptive decision making. In terms of education, women need information about contraceptive mechanisms, health risks, benefits, and side effects to make an informed decision. Contraindications exist to using OCs; however, potential alternatives may exist among other hormonal contraceptives (see Tables 9.4 and 9.5). Side effects of hormonal contraceptives have been reported; however, they are usually temporary and are not serious health risks (see Table 9.6).

One common side effect of lower dose OCs and progestin contraceptives, irregular bleeding, needs to be discussed further. With lower dose pills, breakthrough bleeding and amenorrhea may occur initially and then decrease after continued use (Rosenberg & Long, 1992). There is less occurrence of breakthrough bleeding, spotting, or amenorrhea with multiphasic OCs (Wharton & Blackburn, 1988). Breakthrough bleeding, spotting, and/or amenorrhea are more common with the progestin-only contraceptives (Darney, 1994; Kaunitz, 1994; Liskin & Blackburn, 1987; Stubblefield, 1994).

TABLE 9.4.   Hormonal Contraceptives—Potential Contraindications

Pregnancy
Breast-feeding
Undiagnosed uterine or vaginal bleeding
Recent history of thromboembolism
History of myocardial infarction
Atherosclerosis disease
History of congestive heart failure
Smoker and older than 35 years of age
Hypertension that is difficult to control
Vascular headaches (migraine) with focal symptoms
Headaches (tension or vascular without prior focal symptoms) that increase in severity or frequency
LDL > 190 mg/dl and 0–1 risk factors
LDL > 160 mg/dl and ≥ to 2 risk factors
Diabetes with vascular disease
History of breast cancer
Estrogen dependent neoplasia
Gallbladder disease
Impaired liver function
Renal disease

Sources: Comp & Zacur (1993); Hatcher et al. (1994); Jones & Wild (1994); Knopp et al. (1993); Mattson & Rebar (1993); Mestman & Schmidt-Sarosi (1993); Stenchever (1993); and Sullivan & Lobo (1993).

Information needs to be given verbally as well as in writing at the appropriate reading level. Instructions provided by manufacturers may not be appropriate as reading levels between the 10th and 12th grades may be required (Swanson et al., 1990; Williams-Deane & Potter, 1992), and some instructions may be confusing and inadequate (Williams-Deane & Potter, 1992). Clinic-prepared instructions may be more appropriate than instructions provided by manufacturers; however, clinics need to assess the reading level of their clientele.

After providing information, the risks and benefits need to be discussed in relation to health history and health status. Some hormonal contraceptives may be contraindicated. Once the decision is made, women and their partners need to be provided information on symptoms of potential health risks. They should be encouraged to contact the clinic if any symptoms occur.

The warning signs for oral contraceptives can be remembered by the acronym ACHES as follows (Church & Rinehart [1990]):

TABLE 9.5. Hormonal Contraceptives—Potential Users

Combined OCs

Family history of thrombosis
Using anti-coagulants
Hypertension (controlled) and if young and non-smoker
Tension headaches
Vascular headaches (migraine) without focal symptoms
LDL < 130 mg/dl and 0–1 risk factors
LDL 130–160 mg/dl, 0–1 risk factors, and dietary advice
LDL < 130 mg/dl, ≥ 2 risk factors, > 35 years old
Diabetes without vascular disease
Cervical dysplasia
Benign breast disease
Epilepsy (combined with at least 50 mcg of ethinyl estradiol or
    medroxyprogesterone are best)

Progestin only

Hypertension that is difficult to control
Older in age
Smokers
Atherosclerotic disease
History of thrombosis
Cardiovascular disease and smoking
Diabetic
Breast-feeding
Migraine headaches

Sources: Chi (1993); Comp & Zacur (1993); Darney (1994); Erwin (1994); Hatcher et al. (1994); Jones & Wild (1994); Kaunitz (1994); Knopp et al. (1993); Liskin & Blackburn (1987); Mattson & Rebar (1993); Mestman & Schmidt-Sarosi (1993); Stenchever (1993); Sullivan & Lobo (1993); and Wharton & Blackburn (1988).

A — Severe pain in *abdomen* (stomach)
C — *Chest* pain or problems breathing
H — *Headaches* (more frequent and severe than normal)
E — *Eye* problems (problems seeing)
S — *Swelling* or *severe* pain in a leg

The warning signs for progestin contraceptives are more varied in nature and severity (Hatcher et al., 1994):

Norplant
1. severe lower abdominal pains
2. arm pain

TABLE 9.6. Potential Side Effects of Hormonal Contraceptives

Appearance related
  acne
  alopecia
  hirsutism
  hyperpigmentation over implants
  weight gain
  chloasma

Mood changes
  anxiety
  depression
  nervousness
  reduced libido

Reproductive system related
  irregular menstrual bleeding
  breakthrough bleeding
  spotting
  amenorrhea
  breast tenderness and swelling
  galactorrhea
  leukorrhea
  premenstrual symptoms

Other
  dizziness
  headaches
  nausea
  pruritis
  vomiting

Sources: Darney (1994); Hatcher et al. (1994); Kaunitz (1994); Liskin & Blackburn (1987); Rosenberg & Long (1992); Shoupe & Mishell (1989); Wharton & Blackburn (1988); and Youngkin (1993).

3. heavy bleeding
4. migraine headaches
5. expulsion of implant
6. delayed menstrual periods after being regular
7. pus or bleeding at insertion

Depo-Provera
1. weight gain
2. headaches
3. heavy bleeding

4. depression
5. frequent urination

Mini-pills
abdominal pain

Contraceptive beliefs and attitudes also need to be discussed. Women's attitudes toward oral contraceptives (OCs) and implants have been reported as favorable with more positive attitudes toward OCs than implants (Forrest & Fordyce, 1993). More specific than attitudes are beliefs which also influence contraceptive behavior. For example, predominant reasons for choosing Norplant were more positive beliefs about it in comparison to other methods (Darney et al., 1990; Frank, Poindexter, Johnston, & Bateman, 1992). Beliefs about OCs and Norplant are delineated in Table 9.7. There is a lack of information on women's beliefs about injectables.

OCs and some of the other hormonal methods interact with some medications and vitamins (see Table 9.8). Women need to be instructed to discuss their prescriptions for hormonal contraceptives and other medications with any health professional caring for them. The interaction of OCs and other medications may result in either decreased or increased effectiveness of OCs (Shenfield, 1986). The interaction may be due to a number of mechanisms. For example, there is decreased effectiveness of OCs with some antibiotics as they disrupt the normal bacterial flora in the gastrointestinal tract and thereby decreased absorption of OCs from the gastrointestinal tract (D'Arcy, 1986). There is also decreased effectiveness of OCs with anticonvulsive medications and Rifampicin, which increase metabolism of hormones and their elimination (D'Arcy, 1986). Norplant's effectiveness is also decreased by anticonvulsive medications and Rifampicin (Hatcher et al., 1994). In addition, OCs have the potential to modify a variety of other medications (D'Arcy, 1986; Orme, Back, & Breckenridge, 1983; Shenfield, 1986; Shenfield & Griffin, 1991). For example, OCs enhance the toxicity of imipramine, an antidepressant (D'Arcy, 1986).

However, the risk of pregnancy is reported as low when antibiotics are taken, except for Rifampicin (London & Lookingbull, 1994; Miller, Helms, & Brodell, 1994). Much of the information on drug interactions with hormonal contraceptives is conflicting. It is speculated that the risk of pregnancy from a drug interaction is greatest when a woman has a higher rate of metabolism and is on a low-dose hormonal contraceptive (Fotherby, 1990). It is suggested that breakthrough bleeding may be an indication of OC ineffectiveness when taking other medications (Miller et al., 1994).

TABLE 9.7.   Perceptions of Hormonal Contraceptives

Perceived benefits of OCs
   effective
   convenient
   regulates menses

Perceived barriers of OCs
   unsafe
   expensive
   risk for cancer in general
   risk increased for cardiovascular disease
   risk for fertility problems
   risk for hormonal problems
   risk for headaches or migraines
   risk for weight gain
   no STD protection

Perceived benefits of Norplant
   effectiveness
   safe
   convenient
   less difficult to remember to use than other methods
   no interruption of sex
   long duration of effect
   less worry about pregnancy
   sex more spontaneous

Perceived barriers of Norplant
   side effects
   insertion pain
   menstrual changes and problems
   weight change
   acne
   hormonal effects
   local infection
   headaches

Sources: Darney et al. (1990); Frank, Poindexter, Johnston, & Bateman (1992); Peipert & Gutmann (1993); and Tanfer & Rosenbaum (1986).

ADMINISTRATION OF HORMONAL CONTRACEPTIVES

OCs

It is recommended that low-dose OCs (≤ 35 mcg of estrogen) or prog-estin-only pills be prescribed first (Hatcher et al., 1994). If Rifampicin or anticonvulsive medication is being routinely taken, a 50 mcg dose

TABLE 9.8. Interactions Between Oral Contraceptives and Medications

Decrease effectiveness of OCs: antibiotics, antibacterials, and antifungals

ampicillin	amoxicillin
neomycin	ketoconazole
chloramphenicol	clindamycin
phenoxymethylpenicillin	fluconazole
co-trimoxazole	metronidazole
rifampicin	itraconazole
griseofulvin	cephalexin
tetracycline	terbinafine
isoniazid	dapsone
trimethoprim	telampicillin
erythromycin	minocycline

Antiepilepsy medications

butobarbital	phenobarbital
carbamazepine (Tegretol)	phenytoin (Dilantin)
ethosuximide (Zarontin)	primidone (Mysoline)
mephobarbital	

Analgesics

antipyrine	aspirin
aminopyrine	phenacetin

Nonsteroidal antiinflammatory

phenylbutazone	oxyphenbutazone

Nonbarbiturate hypnotics

dichlorphenazone	meprobamate
glutethimide	

Others

antihistamines/decongestants	dihydroergotamine
chlorpromazine	promethazine (Mepergan, Phenergan)
chlordiazepoxide (Librium)	
diazepam (Valium)	sulfamethoxypyridazine

Increase OCs Concentrations

ascorbic acid

Potentiate side effects of OCs

allopurinol	methandroestenolone
aminosalicylic acid	methylphenidate (Ritalin)
aspirin	MAOI antidepressants
chloramphenicol	phenothiazines
cimetidine (Tagamet)	phenyramidol
disulfiram (Antabuse)	sulfaphenazole
hydrocortisone	triparanol
isoniazid	

Sources: Brodell & Elewski (1995); D'Arcy (1986); London & Lookingbull (1994); Miller, Helms, & Brodell (1994); Orme et al. (1983); Shenfield (1986); and Shenfield & Griffin (1991).

OC may be recommended (Hatcher et al., 1994). After 3 to 6 months, clients should be re-evaluated for any side effects or health risks (Hatcher et al., 1994). Exams become yearly (Hatcher et al., 1994). Adolescents may begin OCs 6 to 12 periods post menarche unless there is a greater pregnancy risk (Hatcher et al., 1994).

In general, hormonal contraceptives are not recommended while breast-feeding. Some recommend progestin-only OCs for women who are breast-feeding as lactation is not inhibited (Wharton & Blackburn, 1988). It is recommended to begin progestin-only OCs after infants are 3 to 4 months old and after menstruation resumes (Wharton & Blackburn, 1988). By waiting, infants are not exposed to trace amounts of hormones found in breast milk during the time of most susceptibility for growth and development and the mother's chance of pregnancy is minimal during the first 6 months postpartum when she is still amenorrheic (Wharton & Blackburn, 1988). However, pharmaceutical companies do not recommend OCs until after weaning the infant/child (PDR, 1995).

Women need to be educated and counseled regarding taking pills (see Table 9.9), missing pills, and skipping menstrual periods. If one combined OC pill is missed, the client should be instructed to immediately take the pill and take the next pill the same time as she usually would (PDR, 1995). The client should be instructed according to the product information for the specific OC if she missed more than one combined OC, one or more progestin-only OC, and if a period was skipped.

A discussion with women about their perceived barriers to using OCs may be beneficial (see Chapter 3). For example, they may perceive that taking OCs will be difficult to remember. Providers may discuss with them ways to remember to take OCs such as associating it with another daily routine such as brushing teeth or eating a meal. Women remembered to take OCs by associating it with a daily routine, having visual reminders, and others reminding them (Balassone, 1989).

Injectables

Injections should be administered during the first 5 days of the menstrual cycle, within the first 5 days following birth in nonbreast-feeding women or after 6 weeks postpartum when breast-feeding (Kaunitz, 1994). After 24 hours of injection, blood levels are sufficient to prevent pregnancy (Kaunitz, 1994). If the first injection is given after the first 5 days of a menstrual period, another method of contraception should be used for 2 weeks (Hatcher et al., 1994).

TABLE 9.9.   Instructions for Taking Combined Oral Contraceptives

How to take birth control pills

1. Begin taking one of 3 ways: (1) the first day of menses, (2) the first Sunday after menses began, or (3) day 5 of menses. Check with the nurse or doctor about which one you should do.

2. Take 1 pill every day.
    a. If you have a 28-pill packet, take 1 each day for 28 days. After taking the last one, begin the next pill packet the next day.
    b. If you have a 21-pill packet, take 1 each day for 21 days. Do not take any pills for the next 7 days. After not taking a pill for 7 days, begin next pill packet.

3. Take each pill at the same time of day.

4. Use another birth control method (condoms, spermicides, or no sex) for the first 7 days of starting birth control pills or if you have vomiting and diarrhea.

5. Do not take a pill at the same time you drink or eat food with vitamin C (orange juice, cantaloupe).

6. Let other health care professionals know that you are taking OCs. OCs may make changes in other medications and laboratory tests.

7. You do not need to take a break from pills for fertility.

8. Call the clinic or talk to the nurse or doctor about any problems you have with the pill.

Progestin only OCs

1. Take 1 pill every day.

2. Take pills at the same time every day.

3. After taking all pills in a packet, start a new packet the next day. Do not take a break between pill packets.

4. Same instructions as combined OCs (#4–#8).

Sources: Chi (1993); Church & Rinehart (1990); Hatcher et al. (1994); *Physicians' Desk Reference* (1995); and Wharton & Blackburn (1988).

Injections are given every 3 months. There is a 2-week period of overlap as it is effective in preventing ovulation for 14 weeks (Kaunitz, 1994). If a woman is 2 weeks or more late for the injection, a negative pregnancy test should be obtained (Kaunitz, 1989).

Administration should be by deep intramuscular injection given with a 21- to 23-gauge needle in the deltoid or gluteus maximus muscle (Hatcher et al., 1994). Effectiveness is decreased by massaging the injection site (Hatcher et al., 1994). Emergency supplies should be available if an allergic reaction to DMPA should occur (Hatcher et al., 1994).

Norplant

Implants are inserted within the first 5 days of the menstrual cycle (Liskin & Blackburn, 1987). If Norplant was not inserted within the first 7 days of the menstrual period, another contraceptive method is needed for the first 24 hours after insertion (Hatcher et al., 1994). Blood levels have the potential to prevent ovulation within 24 hours of insertion (Liskin & Blackburn, 1987). The effects on breast-feeding infants during the first 6 weeks of life is not known, and there has been only one study of the effects on infants beyond 6 weeks (PDR, 1995).

Norplant is inserted and removed through a small incision with local anesthetic (Liskin & Blackburn, 1987) by health care professionals who have special training (Darney, 1994). The implants are inserted under the skin, inside the upper or lower arm (Liskin & Blackburn, 1987). It has been recommended that a pressure dressing be used overnight on the incision to prevent bleeding and steri-strips remain over the incision for 4 days (Shoupe & Mishell, 1989). After 5 years, new implants are inserted when removing old implants, as blood levels are not sufficient to prevent pregnancies beyond 5 years (Darney, 1994).

Insertion and removal of implants have few complications (Liskin & Blackburn, 1987). Bruising and soreness may occur at the site of insertion or removal (Darney, 1994). Rare complications have been reported such as mild itching, scar-tissue formation, hematoma, and infections (Liskin & Blackburn, 1987). Occasionally an implant or piece of one may be difficult to remove (Liskin & Blackburn, 1987).

Although minimal removal complications are noted in the literature, Norplant users perceive problems. There is a class action suit against a manufacturer of Norplant. The basis of the suit is the users' pain and suffering related to removal problems (Contraceptive Technology Update, 1994). It is speculated that publicity about the lawsuit is influential in the increased number of users' requests for Norplant removal and discontinuance (Contraceptive Technology Update, 1995).

EVALUATION

Evaluation should include assessment of safety, side effects, and behaviors that impact effectiveness. Evaluating the safety of hormonal contraceptives involves a reassessment of health status and questioning whether or not any risk symptoms have been experienced, assessment of correct and consistent use of OC pill taking behaviors for OC users, and appointment keeping behavior for users of injectables and implants.

In addition, side effects from hormonal contraceptives need to be assessed (see Table 9.7).

Correct and consistent use of hormonal contraceptives is important. When inconsistent and incorrect use is taken into account, failure rates of 6.2% and 7.3% have been reported for OCs (Jones & Forrest, 1992). In one study, 58% were not consistently taking the pill every day, and 83% were not consistently taking the pill at the same time of day (Oakley & Parent, 1990). When lower dose and progestin-only OCs are missed, hormonal levels may decrease enough to not be effective (Hatcher et al., 1994; Wharton & Blackburn 1988). When appointments are missed for repeat injectables and reinsertion of implants, there is potential for method failure. Therefore, assessment needs to involve behaviors related to correct and consistent use and reasons for not adhering.

Questions to be asked of women might include (Hanna, 1993; Oakley & Parent, 1990):

1. Were pills always taken in the same order?
2. How many pills were left at the end of the month?
3. Was a backup method used if needed?
4. Were pills taken every day?
5. Were pills taken at the same time of day?
6. How were pills taken if one or some were missed?

The following information from the woman's chart should also be assessed. Was a refill prescription appointment made before depletion of the current supply of pills? Did the refill prescription appointment occur before current pills were depleted?

In addition, women's reasons for discontinuance of a method needs to be explored. Of women using hormonal contraceptives, 75% of OCs users, 70% of injection users, and 88% of implant users continue using the method at the end of 1 year (Trussell & Kost, 1987). Stopping the pill occurred after missing pills, running out of supplies, no longer being sexually active (Oakley, Sereika, & Bogue, 1991), and forgetting to take pills (Dinerman, Wilson, Duggan, & Joffe, 1995).

Discontinuance has been reported to be associated with side effects of OCs (Oakley et al., 1991) and Norplant (Darney et al., 1990; Dinerman et al., 1995; Polaneczky et al., 1994). Collaboration on ways to reduce side effects may be beneficial. Taking OCs with food may be suggested when nausea is a problem (Hatcher et al., 1994). Alternative OCs may be tried to reduce side effects. Lower dose estrogen (20 mcg) or progestin-only pills may be tried for nausea, breast tenderness, or vascular headaches, or Ovcon 35, Brevicon, Modicon, Demulin, or new progestin-only pills for acne (Hatcher et al., 1994). If severity and frequency of headaches increase, especially with blurred or lost vision, discontinue the contraceptive (Hatcher et al., 1994). If galactorrhea occurs, other possible reasons (prolactin levels, pregnancy, breast cancer, or suckling the breast during sex) need to be explored (Hatcher et al., 1994).

The side effect of irregular bleeding may need particular attention. Precise definitions are advocated when assessing breakthrough bleeding, which is bleeding other than menstrual, and requiring pads or tampons, and spotting, which does not require pads or tampons (Stubblefield, 1994). When assessing bleeding irregularities, potential causes such as irregular pill taking (Wharton & Blackburn, 1988) and chlamydia infections (Hatcher et al., 1994) need to be considered. If other reasons are ruled out, an increase in estrogen and/or progestin may be recommended to reduce breakthrough bleeding (Hatcher et al., 1994).

SUMMARY

Care for women seeking and using hormonal contraceptives involves assessment, strategies to promote decisions and use, and evaluation. Women's health is assessed along with a health history (with a focus on cardiovascular and reproductive systems). Strategies involve education and counseling regarding risks, benefits, side effects, medication interactions, and contraceptive beliefs. The evaluation phase involves assessing effectiveness, consistent and correct use, and the occurrence of side effects or risk symptoms.

REFERENCES

Althaus F., & Kaeser, L. (1990). At pill's 30th birthday, breast cancer question is unresolved. *Family Planning Perspectives, 22,* 173–176.

Balassone, M. (1989). Risk of contraceptive discontinuation among adolescents. *Journal of Adolescent Health Care, 10,* 527–533.

Brodell, R., & Elewski, B. (1995). Clinical Pearl: Systemic antifungal drugs and drug interactions. *Journal of the American Academy of Dermatology, 33,* 259–260.

Burkman, R. (1994). Noncontraceptive effects of hormonal contraceptives: Bone mass, sexually transmitted disease and pelvic inflammatory disease, cardiovascular disease, menstrual function and future fertility. *American Journal of Obstetrics and Gynecology, 170,* 1569–1575.

Cates, W., & Stone, K. (1992). Family planning, sexually transmitted diseases and contraceptive choice: A literature update—part II. *Family Planning Perspectives, 24,* 122–128.

Chi, I. (1993). The safety and efficacy issues of progestin-only oral contraceptives: An epidemiologic perspective. *Contraception, 47,* 1–21.

Church, C., & Rinehart, W. (1990). Counseling clients about the pill. *Population Reports, 18,* 1–20.

Comp, P., & Zacur, H. (1993). Contraceptive choices in women with coagulation disorders. *American Journal of Obstetrics and Gynecology, 168,* 1990–1993.

Contraceptive Technology Update. (1994). Class-action suit filed against Norplant manufacturer. *Contraceptive Technology Update, 15,* 125–126.

Contraceptive Technology Update. (1995). Pill survey finds OCs still No. 1 choice to manage side effects, cut costs. *Contraceptive Technology Update, 16,* 105–120.

D'Arcy, P. (1986). Drug interactions with oral contraceptives. *Drug Intelligence & Clinical Pharmacy, 20,* 353–362.

Darney, P. (1994). Hormonal implants: contraception for a new century. *American Journal of Obstetrics and Gynecology, 170,* 1536–1543.

Darney, P., Atkinson, E., Tanner, S., MacPherson, S., Hellerstein, S., & Alvarado, A. (1990). Acceptance and perception of Norplant among users in San Francisco, USA. *Studies in Family Planning, 21,* 152–160.

Dinerman, L., Wilson, M., Duggan, A., & Joffe, A. (1995). Outcomes of adolescents using Levonorgestrel implants vs oral contraceptives or other contraceptive methods. *Archives Pediatric Adolescent Medicine, 149,* 967–972.

Erwin, P. (1994). To use or not to use combined hormonal oral contraceptives during lactation. *Family Planning Perspectives, 26,* 26–30, 33.

Forrest, J., & Fordyce, R. (1993). Women's contraceptive attitudes and use in 1992. *Family Planning Perspectives, 25,* 175–179.

Frank, M., Poindexter, A., Johnson, M., & Bateman, L. (1992). Characteristics and attitudes of early contraceptive implant acceptors in Texas. *Family Planning Perspectives, 24,* 208–213.

Fotherby, K. (1990). Interactions with oral contraceptives. *American Journal of Obstetrical Gynecology, 163,* 2153–2159.

Godsland, I., & Crook, D. (1994). Update on the metabolic effects of steroidal contraceptives and their relationship to cardiovascular disease risk. *American Journal of Obstetrics and Gynecology, 170,* 1528–1536.

Godsland, I., Crook, D., & Wynn, V. (1992). Clinical and metabolic considerations of long-term oral contraceptive use. *American Journal of Obstetrics and Gynecology, 166,* 1955–1963.

Grimes, D. (1992). The safety of oral contraceptives: Epidemiologic insights from the first 30 years. *American Journal of Obstetrics and Gynecology, 166,* 1950–1954.

Grimes, D. (1994). The morbidity and mortality of pregnancy: Still risky business. *American Journal of Obstetrics and Gynecology, 170,* 1489–1494.

Hanna, K. (1993). Effect of nurse-client transaction on female adolescents' oral contraceptive adherence. *Image: Journal of Nursing Scholarship, 25,* 285–290.

Hatcher, R., Trussell, J., Stewart, F., Stewart, G., Kowal, D., Guest, F., Cates, W., & Policar, M. (1994). *Contraceptive Technology.* New York: Irvington Publishers.

Herbst, A., & Berek, J. (1993). Impact of contraception on gynecologic cancers. *American Journal of Obstetrics and Gynecology, 168,* 1980–1985.

Jones, E., & Forrest, J. (1992). Contraceptive failure rates based on the 1988 NSFG. *Family Planning Perspectives, 24,* 12–19.

Jones, K. P., & Wild, R. A. (1994). Contraception for patients with psychiatric or medical disorders. *American Journal of Obstetrics and Gynecology, 170,* 1575–1580.

Kaunitz, A. (1989). Injectable contraception. *Clinical Obstetrics and Gynecology, 32,* 356–368.

Kaunitz, A. (1994). Long-acting injectable contraception with depot medroxyprogesterone acetate. *American Journal of Obstetrics and Gynecology, 170,* 1543–1549.

Kennedy, K. (1993). Fertility, sexuality, and contraception during lactation. In J. Riordan & K Auerbach (Eds.), *Breastfeeding and human lactation* (pp. 429–457). Boston: Jones and Bartlett.

Knopp, R., LaRosa, J., & Burkman, R. (1993). Contraception and dyslipidemia. *American Journal of Obstetrics and Gynecology, 168,* 1994–2005.

Liskin, L., & Blackburn, R. (1987). Hormonal contraception: New long-acting methods. *Population Reports, 15,* 57–87.

Liskin, L., & Rutledge, A. (1984). After contraception: Dispelling rumors about later childbearing. *Population Reports, 12,* 697–731.

Lobo, R., & Stanczyk, F. (1994). New knowledge in the physiology of hormonal contraceptives. *American Journal of Obstetrics and Gynecology, 170,* 1499–1507.

London, B., & Lookingbull, D. (1994). Frequency of pregnancy in acne patients taking oral antibiotics and oral contraceptives. *Archives of Dermatology, 130,* 392–393.

McGregor, J., & Hammill, H. (1993). Contraception and sexually transmitted diseases: Interactions and opportunities. *American Journal of Obstetrics and Gynecology, 168,* 2033–2041.

Mattson, R., & Rebar, R. (1993). Contraceptive methods for women with neurologic disorders. *American Journal of Obstetrics and Gynecology, 168,* 2027–2032.

Mestman, J., & Schmidt-Sarosi, C. (1993). Diabetes mellitus and fertility control: Contraception management issues. *American Journal of Obstetrics and Gynecology, 168,* 2012–2020.

Miller, D., Helms, S., & Brodell, R. (1994). A practical approach to antibiotic treatment in women taking oral contraceptives. *Journal of the American Academy of Dermatology, 30,* 1008–1011.

Mishell, D. (1993). Noncontraceptive benefits of oral contraceptives. *Journal of Reproductive Medicine, 38,* 1021–1029.

Mosher, W. (1990). Contraceptive practice in the United States, 1982–1988. *Family Planning Perspectives, 22,* 198–205.

Oakley, D., & Parent, J. (1990). A scale to measure microbehaviors of oral contraceptive pill use. *Social Biology, 37,* 215–222.

Oakley, D., Sereika, S., & Bogue, E. (1991). Oral contraceptive pill use after an initial visit to a family planning clinic. *Family Planning Perspectives, 23,* 150–154.

Orme, M., Back, D., & Breckenridge, A. (1983). Clinical phamacokinetics of oral contraceptive steroids. *Clinical Pharmacokinetics, 8,* 95–136.

Peipert, J., & Gutmann, J. (1993). Oral contraceptive risk assessment: A survey of 247 educated women. *Obstetrics & Gynecology, 82,* 112–117.

Physicians' Desk Reference. (49th ed.). (1995). Montvale, NJ: Medical Economics Data Production Co.

Polaneczky, M., Slap, G., Forke, C., Rappaport, A., & Sondheimer, S. (1994). The use of levonorgestrel implants (Norplant) for contraception in adolescent mothers. *New England Journal of Medicine, 331,* 1201–1206.

Rosenberg, M., & Long, S. (1992). Oral contraceptives and cycle control: A critical review of the literature. *Advances in Contraception, 8,* 35–45.

Samsioe, G. (1994). Coagulation and anticoagulation effects of contraceptive steroids. *American Journal of Obstetrics and Gynecology, 170,* 1523–1527.

Shenfield, G. (1986). Drug interactions with oral contraceptive preparations. *Medical Journal of Australia, 144,* 205–211.

Shenfield, G., & Griffin, J. (1991). Clinical pharmacokinetics of contraceptive steroids: An update. *Clinical Pharmacokinetics, 20,* 15–37.

Shoupe, D., & Mishell, D. (1989). Norplant: Subdermal implant system for long-term contraception. *American Journal of Obstetrics and Gynecology, 160,* 1286–1292.

Stenchever, M. (1993). Risks of oral contraceptive use in women over 35. *Journal of Reproductive Medicine, 38,* 1030–1035.

Stubblefield, P. (1994). Menstrual impact of contraception. *American Journal of Obstetrics and Gynecology, 170,* 1513–1522.

Sullivan, J., & Lobo, R. (1993). Considerations for contraception in women with cardiovascular disorders. *American Journal of Obstetrics and Gynecology, 168,* 2006–2011.

Swanson, J., Forrest, K., Ledbetter, C., Hall, S., Holstine, E., & Shafer, M. (1990). Readability of commercial and generic contraceptive instructions. *IMAGE: Journal of Nursing Scholarship, 22,* 96–100.

Tanfer, K., & Rosenbaum, E. (1986). Contraceptive perceptions and method choice among young single women in the United States. *Studies in Family Planning, 17,* 269–277.

Trussell, J., & Kost, K. (1987). Contraceptive failure in the United States: A critical review of the literature. *Studies in Family Planning, 18,* 237–283.

Wharton, C. & Blackburn, R. (1988). Lower-dose pills. *Population Reports, 16,* 1–31.

Williams-Deane, M., & Potter, L. (1992). Current oral contraceptive use instructions: An analysis of patient package inserts. *Family Planning Perspectives, 24,* 111–115.

Youngkin, E. (1993). Progestogens: A look at the "other" hormone. *Nurse Practitioner, 18,* 28–40.

Female Barrier Methods of Contraception

Joyce E. White

Although the development of more effective birth control methods whose use is not related to coitus has eclipsed the use of female barrier methods, these methods continue to play an important role in contraception in the United States. Currently, use of female barrier methods is directly associated with age of the user. Although only 0.8% of women aged 15 to 19 who were at risk of pregnancy reported using the diaphragm in the 1988 National Survey of Family Growth (N.S.F.G.), 7.3% of those aged 35 to 39 did so (Mosher & Pratt, 1990). Recent indications that female dependent barrier methods provide protection at least as strong as that afforded by condoms against certain sexually transmitted diseases (Rosenberg et al., 1992) may increase the use of these methods and spur the development of new approaches.

HISTORY OF FEMALE BARRIER METHODS OF CONTRACEPTION

The use of female barriers, like that of male sheaths, began in ancient times. Ancient Egyptian writings, the Papyrus Ebers, contained a prescription for a method that involved moistening lint with a concoction of a mixture of drugs and honey and placing it against the mouth of the uterus (Papyrus Ebers, c. 1550 BC). This represents only one of a number of occlusive devices that have been used over the centuries, perhaps the most famous of which is half a squeezed lemon, whose use is attributed to the noted 18th century lover, Casanova (Chalker, 1987).

THE ROLE OF THE CLINICIAN IN PROVIDING
FEMALE BARRIER METHODS

Because, to a large extent, clinicians may be viewed as gatekeepers to women's access to contraception, especially where the method requires a prescription or clinical services (Lethbridge, 1990; Russell & Love, 1991), it is important that they recognize their own attitudes toward a variety of contraceptive options and that they are consistent in providing accurate information. A study conducted a number of years ago discovered that clinic personnel were citing lowest reported failure rates for oral contraceptives and IUDs and typical failure rates for diaphragms (Trussell, Faden, & Hatcher, 1976). Table 8.2 in Chapter 8 shows the effectiveness of female barrier methods and compares it to the use of no contraceptive method. It demonstrates the relationship of parity to the effectiveness of certain methods, notably the cervical cap.

In counseling individuals about female barriers of contraception, clinicians need to explore the acceptability of a method and give accurate information on which clients can make informed decisions. This may involve exploring the details of individuals' sexual activity because frequency of intercourse, patterns of intercourse (throughout the week or during infrequent visits of sexual partners), and need for protection against sexually transmitted diseases may all influence the contraceptive choice.

Clinicians also need to analyze their own characteristics and the characteristics of their practice. Do they have the interest in doing the patient education, which is part of providing female barrier methods of contraception? Does the physical setup allow women the time they need in practicing with a method in order to gain dexterity or will someone be knocking on the examining room door every 5 minutes inquiring if the patient is "finished yet"? Do they provide contraceptive services frequently enough to maintain a level of expertise in fitting devices such as diaphragms and cervical caps?

All female barrier methods have the following advantages. They are under the control of the woman alone and do not require partner involvement. They do not cause systemic side effects and do not alter women's hormonal patterns. They are especially attractive for women who need protection intermittently. They provide protection immediately upon use.

Because the use of barrier methods is related to coitus with the perception of loss of spontaneity, consistent use has been found to be a problem with many failures being "user failures" rather than "method failures." A major disadvantage common to female barrier methods is the alteration in vaginal flora associated with spermicides, either alone or in combination with physical barriers, which apparently causes a shift in vaginal flora supporting the growth of pathogens, resulting in vaginal candidiasis or bacterial vaginosis (Hooten et al., 1991). Toxic shock syndrome is also a potential side effect of the diaphragm or cervical cap, although the magnitude of this risk is said to be low (Hatcher et al., 1994). For this reason these methods are not recommended for use during menses.

THE METHODS

The following section describes each of the female barrier methods, reviewing advantages and disadvantages of each, as well as recommended patient education. It also reviews fitting procedures for those devices, which require fitting by clinicians.

CHEMICAL BARRIERS: FOAMS, GELS, SUPPOSITORIES, FILM

These chemical barriers have in common the presence of two components: nonoxynol-9, which serves as a chemical to kill sperm, and a delivery system for the nonoxynol-9. Nonoxynol-9 is the most commonly used spermicide in the world. A surface surfactant, nonoxynol-9 damages the cell walls of sperm, and a number of studies indicate that it damages the cell walls of many pathogens, including *Neisseria gonorrhoea, Trichomonas vaginalis, Herpes simplex* virus, *Treponema pallidum,* and *Ureaplasma urealyticum,* as well, leading to a reduction in sexually transmitted diseases among those who use them (Amortegui et al., 1984). While some studies have found nonoxynol-9 to also be effective against *Chlamydia trachomatis* (Benes & McCormack, 1985), others have not (Kappus & Quinn, 1986).

Concerns have been raised about the possibility that nonoxynol-9 might, in spite of its ability to disrupt the cell membranes of pathogens which cause sexually transmitted diseases, be harmful in high doses. One study found nonoxynol-9 delivered via vaginal sponge to be associated with higher rates of HIV seroconversion (Kreiss et al., 1992). It is speculated that this may result from the same membrane-disrupting effect on vaginal mucosa that make this chemical an effective bacteriocidal and spermicidal agent (Cates & Stone, 1992).

Spermicides can be used alone, but are also frequently recommended for use with physical barriers, including diaphragms, cervical caps, and condoms. The combination of spermicide and physical barrier has been found to greatly increase contraceptive effectiveness. One investigator found condoms used alone to result in a 3% failure rate, spermicide alone in a 6% failure rate, and condoms and spermicide used together in only a 0.01% failure rate (Kestelman & Trussell, 1991).

Description

Vaginal spermicides are available as foam, gels and creams, suppositories, and film. It is impossible to make meaningful comparisons between one spermicidal preparation and another. Consistency of use and attending to the onset and length of contraceptive protection are probably more important than the delivery system itself (Hatcher et al., 1994). Table 10.1 describes these time intervals.

Advantages

Vaginal spermicides can be obtained without a prescription. They can be used to enhance the effectiveness of other methods, and they reduce the transmission of organisms that cause many sexually transmitted diseases.

Disadvantages

Some delivery systems, notably suppositories and film, require a waiting period before they are effective. The taste of vaginal spermicides is unpleasant, interfering with oral sex, and allergy or sensitivity either to the base or to the nonoxynol-9 itself may develop.

Patient Education

Patients should be instructed to use spermicide each time they have coitus, to insert the spermicide before there is any penetration, and to add an additional application if more than one hour has elapsed between insertion and intercourse.

THE DIAPHRAGM

Description

The diaphragm is a dome-shaped rubber cup that is designed to fit snugly under the cervix in the posterior vaginal fornix, while its anterior rim fits in the notch behind the pubic bone. Thus, it covers not only

TABLE 10.1.   Spermicides with Onset of Action and Length of Effectiveness

Delivery system	Onset of action	Length of time effective
Film	15 minutes	No more than 1 hour
Foam	Immediately	At least 1 hour
Jellies/creams	Immediately	At least 1 hour
Suppositories	15 minutes	No more than 1 hour

the cervix and its os, but the anterior vaginal wall as well. Diaphragms are available in three rim types—arcing spring, coil spring, and flat spring; in two rim widths—conventional and wide seal, and in sizes ranging from 50 mm to 105 mm in diameter.

Advantages

The diaphragm is equally effective in both multiparous and nulliparous women and, when used as directed with a spermicide, it has been found to decrease transmission of STDs. Diaphragm users have lower rates of cervical cancer than do all women, oral contraceptive, and IUD users (Celentano et al., 1987; Vessey, 1978).

Disadvantages

Rates of urinary tract infections are higher among diaphragm users perhaps both as a result of alteration in vaginal flora and trauma during intercourse from the diaphragm's rim. Some women, especially those using the firmer arcing spring diaphragm, experience discomfort during the 6 to 8 hours after coitus that the diaphragm must be left in place. The need to add extra spermicide for subsequent acts of intercourse if they occur within that 6- to 8-hour period causes an uncomfortably wet sensation, which many women find unpleasant. Some women may become allergic to the latex from which the diaphragm is manufactured.

Patient Education

Patients should be instructed to insert the diaphragm no more than 6 hours before intercourse, to leave it in place for 8 hours after intercourse, and to always use it together with a chemical spermicide. After the diaphragm is inserted, its placement should be evaluated by feeling that the back rim of the diaphragm is tucked under the cervix, and the front rim behind the pubic bone. The cervix should be felt through the diaphragm, which is covering it completely. The diaphragm should not be left in place longer than 24 hours and the use of oil-based vaginal medications or lubricants should be avoided as they may cause deterioration of the latex. The diaphragm should be washed with soap and water, thoroughly dried after each use, and should not be stored in bright sunlight.

Following are directions for diaphragm fitting.

- Use fitting diaphragms, not fitting rings, so that both the rim type and size are correct.
- Always have the woman practice insertion and removal before leaving with a diaphragm prescription. Check the correctness of placement before the woman finishes practicing.
- Be sure to scrupulously clean and disinfect the fitting diaphragms between women. (Wash with soap and water and then completely immerse in 60% isopropyl alcohol or its equivalent for 30 minutes.)
- To select a rim type evaluate the depth of the pubic notch, the position of the cervix, and the competence of the vaginal musculature. (Almost all women can be fit with the arcing spring diaphragm and it is easiest to learn to insert. However, this rim type is most likely to cause cramping and discomfort during wear following coitus. For that reason, the coil spring may be the best choice when its use can be mastered by the woman and when there is adequate vaginal muscle tone. The flat rim is best in the woman with adequate vaginal muscle tone and a shallow pubic notch.)
- To determine the correct size:
  1. Insert the first two fingers into the vagina until the middle finger is in the posterior fornix.
  2. Use your thumb to mark the point at which your index finger touches the pubic bone.
  3. After removing your fingers try fitting diaphragms against the end of your middle finger and the spot marked on your index finger until you find one that matches up. (After a few opportunities to fit diaphragms, you will be able to make a good guess without needing to do this.)
  4. Insert the diaphragm you have selected and evaluate its fit. There should be just enough space to place a finger tip between the anterior rim of the diaphragm and the pubic bone and the posterior rim should be snugly in the posterior vaginal fornix.
  5. Remember that the vaginal depth increases during sexual

arousal and the diaphragm should be large enough to account for this; a diaphragm that is just barely large enough in the exam room will probably be too small and may move out of place during coitus.

THE CERVICAL CAP

Description

Chalker (1987) has written, "The existence of the cervical cap is surely one of the best-kept secrets of the twentieth century"(p. 1). Although there are probably about six styles of cervical caps manufactured today, only the Prentif cavity rim cervical cap, manufactured by Lamberts (Dalston) Ltd. of London is approved for use in the United States. It resembles a large thimble, has a soft latex dome and a firm rim. Available in only four sizes, it is designed to fit only over the cervix rather than, as does the diaphragm, covering the entire anterior vaginal wall.

Advantages

The cervical cap, because it is not dependent on the vaginal musculature to keep it in place, can be fit even in the presence of lax vaginal muscle tone. The small size of the cap and its deep dome requires less spermicide, and the spermicide that is used is less likely to be smeared on the vulva when the cap is being placed. Also, because most clinicians recommend that the cap be left in place for up to 3 days and do not recommend the use of additional spermicide for repeated acts of intercourse, the cap is less "messy." (It should be noted, however, that the manufacturer recommends that the cap be left in place no longer than 24 hours and that additional spermicide be inserted in the vagina for additional acts of intercourse.)

Disadvantages

Few clinicians offer the cervical cap as part of their practices and some clinicians have literally never seen a cervical cap. Because only one rim type, available in only four sizes, is approved by the FDA, many women who wish to use the cap cannot be fit satisfactorily. Some sexual partners complain of discomfort during coitus and the cap can be dislodged during coitus. Finally, odor is a frequently reported problem and is directly associated with the length of time that the cap is left in place.

Patient Education

Patients should be instructed to feel for their cervix before inserting the cap and then to be sure that the cap covers the cervix after it is inserted. The cap should always be used with a spermicide, can be placed several hours or at least ½ hour before intercourse, and should be left in place for 8 hours after intercourse. During the first few acts of intercourse in a different coital position, condoms should also be used to assure that this position is not associated with cap dislodgment. Never use the cap with oil-based vaginal medication or lubricant. After each use wash the cap with soap and water and if odor develops try alternating the use of two or three caps or soak the cap for a few minutes in diluted lemon juice, vinegar, rubbing alcohol, bleach, or hydrogen peroxide.

Directions for fitting cervical caps follow.

- After the cap size has been selected and fit evaluated, have the woman spend 20 to 30 minutes with the cap in place and then recheck the fit before proceeding with having her practice.
- Always have the woman practice insertion and removal before leaving with a cervical cap. Check the correctness of placement before the woman finishes practicing.
- Be sure to scrupulously clean and disinfect the fitting caps between patients. (Wash with soap and water and then completely immerse in 60% isopropyl alcohol or its equivalent for 30 minutes.)
- To determine the correct size:
  - The cervix should be positioned in the same plane as the vagina; that is, it should not be at an angle as is usually the case with an extremely anteverted or retroverted uterus. Although caps may fit when the cervix is located at an angle, dislodgment is more common because during intercourse the penis strikes the side of the cap rather than its dome.
  - The cervical walls should be long enough so that the rim can be held in place with a suction action. Cervical walls that are too shallow do not accommodate the Prentif Cavity Rim cap well.
  - When checking for fit, the following maneuvers are useful: Check for evidence of suction by determining the cap's resistance to being pulled off the cervix. Try rotating the cap on the cervix; it should not rotate easily or slip off when it is being rotated. Sweep your finger around the entire cap rim, checking for gaps and attempt to dislodge the cap by gently probing the rim.

THE FEMALE CONDOM

Until recently the only condom available to women in the United States has been the male condom (although a vaginal sheath was used during the early part of this century in Europe, intended for women whose partners were infected with STDs and who were, therefore, at risk for contracting these diseases while performing their "conjugal duties"). The female condom now available is seen as providing important protection against STDs, especially HIV, while providing contraceptive protection as well.

Description

The currently available female condom is a vaginal pouch made of polyurethane with rings at both ends. The ring on the closed end is designed to fit high in the vagina and anchor the condom. The ring at the open end rests on the perineum, anchoring the device during intercourse. The interior surface of the condom is prelubricated with a silicon-based lubricant.

Advantages

The female condom theoretically provides the same protection against STDs as does the male condom, but removes the necessity of negotiating with one's partner about condom use. It is available over the counter. In vitro testing has shown the female condom to be an effective barrier to HIV.

Disadvantages

Some users have reported slippage of the device during intercourse and the female condom at over $8.00 each is more expensive than the male condom.

Patient Education

A new condom must be used for each act of intercourse. The condom can be inserted immediately or up to 8 hours before intercourse, The inner ring must be pushed high into the vagina with about 1 inch of the open end outside the body and the outer ring resting on the lips of the vagina. After intercourse the condom must be removed immediately, being careful to squeeze and twist the outer ring to keep semen inside of the pouch.

SUMMARY

Female barrier methods of contraception, while providing only a small fraction of the contraception practiced in the United States, are seen as playing an increasingly important role, not only in pregnancy protection, but in STD prevention as well. Margaret Sanger, jailed and vilified for her contraceptive work in the early part of this century, wrote:

> It seems inartistic and sordid to insert a pessary or a suppository in anticipation of the sexual act. But it is far more sordid to find yourself several years later burdened down with half a dozen unwanted children, helpless, starved, shoddily clothed, dragging at your skirt, yourself a dragged out shadow of the woman you once were. (Margaret Sanger in Family Limitation, as quoted in Hatcher et al., 1994)

REFERENCES

Amortegui, A., Melder, R., Meyer, M., & Singh, B. (1984). The effect of chemical intravaginal contraceptives and betadine on ureaplasma urealyticum. *Contraception, 30,* 135–137.

Benes, S., & McCormack, W. (1985). Inhibition of growth of chlamydia trachomatis by nonoxynol-9 in vitro. *Antimicrobial Agents and Chemotherapy, 27,* 724–726.

Cates, W., & Stone, K. (1992). Family planning, sexually transmitted diseases and contraceptive choice: A literature update—part 1. *Family Planning Perspectives, 24,* 75–84.

Chalker, R. (1987). *The complete cervical cap guide.* New York: Harper and Row.

Hatcher, R., Trussell, J., Stewart, F., Stewart, G., Kowal, D., Guest, F., Cates, W., & Policar, M. (1994). *Contraceptive technology,* (16th ed.). New York: Irvington Publishers.

Hooten, T. M., Hillier, S., Johnson, C., Roberts, A. L., & Stamm, W. E. (1991). Escherichia coli bacteriuria and contraceptive method. *Journal of the American Medical Association, 265,* 64–69.

Kappus, E., & Quinn, T. (1986). The spermicide nonoxynol-9 does not inhibit chlamydia trachomatis in vitro. *Sexually Transmitted Diseases, 13,* 134–137.

Kestelman, P., & Trussell, J. (1991). Efficacy of the simultaneous use of condoms and spermicides. *Family Planning Perspectives, 23,* 226–227.

Kreiss, J., Ngugi, E., Holmes, K., Ndinya-Achola, J., Waiyaki, P., Roberts, P., Ruminjo, I., Sajabi, R., Kimata, J., Fleming, T., Anzala A., Holton, D., & Plummer, F. (1992). Efficacy of nonoxynol-9 contraceptive sponge use in preventing heterosexual acquisition of HIV in Nairobi prostitutes. *Journal of the American Medical Association, 268,* 477–482.

Lethbridge, D. J. (1990). Women's experience with contraception. Towards a theory of contraceptive self-care. *Nursing Research, 40,* 276–280.

Mosher, W. D., & Pratt, W. F. (1990). Contraceptive use in the United States, 1973–1988. *Advance data from vital and health statistics, No. 182.* Hyattsville, MD: National Center for Health Statistics.

Papyrus Ebers (c. 1550) *Pl. 93,* 6–8.

Rosenberg, M., Davison, A., Jian-Hua C., Judson, F., & Douglas, J. (1992). Barrier contraceptives and sexually transmitted diseases in women: A comparison of female-dependent methods and condoms. *American Journal of Public Health, 82,* 669–674.

Russell, M., & Love, E. (1991) Contraceptive prescription: Physician beliefs, attitudes and socio-demographic characteristics. *Canadian Journal of Public Health, 28,* 259–262.

Trussell, J., Faden, R., & Hatcher, R. (1976). Efficacy information in contraceptive counseling: those little white lies. *American Journal of Public Health, 66,* 761–767.

Vessey, M. (1978). Contraceptive methods: Risks and benefits. *British Medical Journal, 2,* 721–722.

CHAPTER ELEVEN

The Male Barrier Method: Condoms

Kathleen M. Hanna

C ondoms provide a physical barrier for preventing pregnancy and sexually transmitted diseases (STDs). The physical barrier prevents direct contact between the penis and vagina, and cervix, or anus, and it is impermeable to sperm and many pathogenic organisms (Cates & Stone, 1992; Lisken, Wharton, & Blackburn, 1990). In addition, condoms prelubricated with spermicides provide a chemical as well as a physical barrier. Spermicides are surfactants that inactivate sperm and pathogenic organisms by damaging cell walls (Cates & Stone, 1992). Nonoxynol-9 is the predominate spermicide in the United States (Cates & Stone, 1992).

ASSESSMENT

An assessment of factors associated with condom use, health risks, potential benefits and side effects follows. Knowledge of men and women's condom use and associated factors helps screen for those who may be at greater risk for nonuse. Health risks or side effects may be contraindications, whereas potential benefits may be reasons for using condoms.

Factors to consider include:

- *Risk Screening*
  female
  older
  no use or inconsistent use in the past
  one or many sexual partners
  alcohol or drug use
- *Health Risks and Contraindications*
  allergy to latex
- *Benefits of Using Condoms*
  effective in preventing pregnancy
  protection from STDs
  decrease sperm allergy
  decrease premature ejaculation
  minimal expense
  accessible
  lack of side effects

CONDOM USE

Condom use differs among various populations (see Tables 11.1 & 11.2). More males than females currently use condoms. Condom use is considerably higher for partners of adolescent than adult females and slightly higher for adolescent than adult males. In addition, condom rates differ among samples from various high-risk groups.

Condom use varies with number and type of sexual partners and this seems to be a complex relationship. Condom use is less for those with one partner or regular partners and for those with the greatest number of partners or casual partners. Perhaps low condom use is related to low perceived risk for STDs as in the case for those with one or a regular partner. Perhaps risk-taking behavior is a stronger influence for low condom use among those with the greatest number of partners. Risk taking behavior has been associated with high-risk sexual behavior (Jemmott & Jemmott, 1993; Keller et al., 1991; Orr & Langefeld, 1993).

Condom use rates vary in terms of how and when they are measured. For example, rates for "condom use" are greater than for "condoms are always used." Rates also vary in terms of whether they are used alone or with another contraceptive method. Perhaps this is associated with the reason for using condoms—prevention of pregnancy, STDs, or HIV. In addition, condom use has been increasing which is most likely related to the AIDS epidemic.

TABLE 11.1.　Rates of Condom Use Among National Samples

Condom use measured as:	Year and percentage		Sample	Study
Currently using	1982	1988		N.S.F.G.
	12	15	• 15–44-year-old females	Mosher, 1990
	21	33	• 15–19-year-old females	
Currently using	1987	1992		Ortho Birth
	17	25	• 15–44-year-old females	Control Study,
	15	19	• those married	Forrest &
	18	33	• those not married	Fordyce (1993)
Currently using	1988–89			N.S.F.G. &
• condoms only	11		• 15–44-year-old females	General Social
• condoms with other methods	8			Survey, Kost & Forrest (1992)
• prevention of pregnancy	9			
• for prevention of STD/HIV	7			
• for prevention of pregnancy and STD/HIV	4			
Condom alone or with other contraception	1988 53	1991 56	• 17–19-year-old males	National Survey of Adolescent Men, Pleck, Sonenstein, & Ku (1993)
Currently using	1991 51		• 20–39-year-old males	National Survey of Men, Grady, Klepinger, Billy, & Tanfer (1993)
Used with last sexual inter- course	1992		• 12–19-year-olds who have not completed high school	Youth Risk Behavior Survey CDC (1994)
	60		• in school	
	50		• out of school	

TABLE 11.2. Examples of Condom Use Among Various Samples

Condom use measured as:	Percentage	Characteristics of sample	Study
Always used		Females < 45 years old who were HIV infected or at risk for HIV	Galavotti & Schnell (1994)
• condoms only	43		
• BCP only	22		
• both	11		
Always used		Census tracts with high rates of STDs and drug programs, San Francisco, 20–44 years	Catania et al., (1992)
	9	• heterosexual males and females	
	48	• homosexual and bisexual males	
Always used in the past year		Statewide survey of 16–19 year olds in MA	Hingson, Strunin, Berlin, & Heeren (1990)
	29	• 1 partner	
	36	• 2–4 partners	
	26	• 5–9 partners	
	17	• ≥ 10 partners	
Always used		Intravenous drug users, NYC males	CDC (1992)
	33	• with regular partner	
	19	• with casual partner	
Always used in past 30 days		STD Clinics in Denver, Newark, Long Beach, and San Francisco	CDC (1993)
	14	• females with regular partner	
	29	• females with casual partner	
	21	• males with regular partner	
	31	• males with casual partner	
Always used		7–9th graders who had had sexual intercourse, ethnically diverse, from an inner city, California	DiClemente et al. (1992)
	50	• with 1 partner	
	39	• with 2 partners	
	27	• with ≥ 3 partners	

HEALTH RISKS AND CONTRADICTIONS

An uncommon health risk is an allergic reaction to latex condoms (Billow, 1992).

BENEFITS

Effective

Condoms are effective in preventing pregnancies and STDs. When used correctly and consistently, the failure rate in preventing pregnancies is 2% for condoms alone (Trussell & Kost, 1987) and is .05% for condoms combined with spermicides (Kestelman & Trussell, 1991). Taking into account incorrect and inconsistent use, the failure rate in preventing pregnancies is 16% (Jones & Forrest, 1992). The failure rate in preventing STDs is 2% for condoms, 5% for spermicides, and 0.1% for condoms combined with spermicides (Kestelman & Trussell, 1991). The efficacy of the polyurethane condom to prevent pregnancy and STDs is not known (Contraceptive Technology Update, 1995a).

Effectiveness is partially dependent upon condom quality, which is controlled by the U.S. Food and Drug Administration (Cates & Stone, 1992). The standard for condom integrity does not allow greater than 4 failures per 1,000 (Billow, 1992). Condom integrity is tested by filling condoms with 300 ml of water and examining for leaks (Vinson & Epperly, 1991). Air-burst and stretch tests are also performed by manufacturers to ensure quality (Vinson & Epperly, 1991). The polyurethane condom is currently being tested. Areas to be addressed in the testing are prevention of pregnancy and STDs, possibility of toxicity, durability with oil-based products and spermicides, and slippage and breakage rates (Contraceptive Technology Update, 1995a, 1995b).

Sexual Pleasure

Premature ejaculation may be prevented as condoms decrease stimulation (Vinson & Epperly, 1991).

Sperm Allergy

Condoms decrease allergic reactions to semen or sperm among women so predisposed (Hatcher et al., 1994).

Sexually Transmitted Diseases

Condoms provide protection from some STDs. In a review of studies conducted in laboratories, findings support that latex condoms are not permeable to herpes simplex virus, chlamydia, cytomegalovirus, and human immunodeficiency virus (HIV) (Cates & Stone, 1992). Natural membrane condoms are permeable to HIV and herpes simplex virus (Cates & Stone, 1992). In addition, findings from a review of epidemiological and experimental studies support that condoms provide protection from gonorrhea and ureaplasma urealyticum for males (Cates & Stones, 1992). However, for females, the studies are not as conclusive (Cates & Stone, 1992). For females who had used condoms, there was a decreased risk of herpes simplex, genital ulcers, gonorrhea, trichomoniasis, and HIV while they did not have a reduced risk for chlamydia, human papillomavirus, and bacterial vaginosis (Cates & Stone, 1992). Preexisting genital lesions may have affected these findings as protection from STDs is not sufficient when condoms do not cover genital lesions (Lisken et al., 1990).

Condoms prelubricated with spermicides provide further protection from STDs. In a review of studies conducted in laboratories, findings support that spermicides inactivate gonorrhea, trichomoniasis, herpes simplex virus, HIV, treponema pallidum, and ureaplasma urealyticum (Cates & Stone, 1992). It is inconclusive whether or not spermicides inactivate chlamydia in laboratory studies (Cates & Stone, 1992). In addition, findings from review of epidemiological and experimental studies support that spermicides provide protection from gonorrhea, chlamydia, trichomoniasis, and bacterial vaginosis (Cates & Stone, 1992). However, there was not any reduced risk for human papillomavirus, herpes simplex, escherichia coli, and genital ulcers (Cates & Stone, 1992).

There is some recent concern about nonoxynol-9. In a review of the few studies conducted, it is inconclusive whether or not nonoxynol-9 damages genital and rectal epithelium cells (Bird, 1991). It is speculated that if nonoxynol-9 damages cells, these cells may be a potential entry site for HIV (Bird, 1991).

Condom and spermicide use decreases the risk for other female reproductive conditions that are associated with STDs. Women's risk of pelvic inflammatory disease decreases with the use of condoms and spermicides (Cates & Stone, 1992). In addition, use of condoms decreases the risk of ectopic pregnancy and cervical cancer in women (Lisken et al., 1990).

Assessable

A broad and diverse choice of condoms exists with greater than 100 brands that differ in shape, color, scent, texture, lubrication, and reservoir tip (Hatcher et al., 1994). The majority are latex and the minority are natural condoms, which are made from lambs' intestines (Hatcher et al., 1994). Recently, a polyurethane condom, the Avanti, is being marketed in a limited number of states in the United States (Contraceptive Technology Update, 1995b). The average condom is 170 mm in length, 50 mm in width, and .03 to .10 mm in thickness (Hatcher et al., 1994).

Expense

Condoms are one of the least expensive contraceptive methods. Gold Circle Coin is one of the least expensive (with one of the lowest failure rates), while Mentor is one of the most expensive (Consumer Reports, 1989).

Lack of Side Effects

Side effects have not been reported with condoms (Vinson & Epperly, 1991).

STRATEGIES FOR INTERVENTION

Education and counseling men and women about condom use is advocated. They need to be educated on condom use in terms of why, when, and how to use. Information needs to be provided on the effectiveness in preventing unintended pregnancies, STDs, and HIV. In addition, information should include how to use them consistently and correctly to be effective. Provision of written and verbal instructions are suggested. Instructions need to be at an appropriate reading level (Steiner et al., 1993). In addition to education, providers may collaborate with men and women in their decision to use condoms. In this process, condom risks, benefits, and beliefs need to be discussed.

Teaching about condoms should include common "do's and don'ts" as well as when and how to use them. Do's and don'ts include (Billow, 1992; Hatcher et al., 1994; Lisken et al., 1990; Vinson & Epperly, 1991):

Do's
1. Have condoms available before there is a need.
2. Keep condoms in a cool place out of light. Condoms may tear and break more easily if exposed to heat, light, and humidity.
3. Be careful as fingernails and rings may tear condoms or damage packages.
4. Keep nonoil-based lubricant and spermicide on hand.

Don'ts
1. Do not reuse a condom.
2. Do not use the condom if:
   - the package is damaged in any way
   - the date on the package states it was made more than five years ago
   - the condom's color has changed or is uneven
   - the condom is brittle, sticky, or dry
   - the condom is torn
3. If unrolled onto the penis incorrectly, do not try to reroll and use it (woman could be exposed to fluids from the penis that were on the inside of the condom when unrolled one way and now on the outside of the condom when unrolled the other way).
4. Do not unroll a condom prior to putting it on and do not test a condom for holes or leaks (the manufacturer has already done this).

Instructions regarding when and how to use condoms include (Billow, 1992; Hatcher et al., 1994; Lisken et al., 1990; Vinson & Epperly, 1991):

When to Use
1. Use a condom every time you have sexual intercourse.
2. Put a condom on the penis when erect, prior to its touching the partner.

How to Use
1. Squeeze air out of the tip with fingers (this leaves an empty space and may decrease breakage) and hold the condom with the rolled rim on the outside.
2. Hold onto the tip and unroll onto the penis all the way down to the base of the penis (you do not need to stretch the condom). You or your partner may put it on together.
3. If you wish, use a water-based lubricant (K-Y jelly, glycerin, or egg white).
4. If you wish, use a spermicide (nonoxynol-9) for more protection.
5. Withdraw the penis after ejaculation and while the penis is still hard. Hold the condom at the base of the penis while withdrawing.
6. Remove the condom from the penis away from the partner and be careful not to spill semen.
7. Look at the condom for any tears or holes.
8. Throw the used condom into the garbage.
9. If a condom tears or slips off, use foam spermicide immediately or wash the penis and vagina with soap and water if a spermi-

cide is not available. See your health care provider about preventing pregnancy.

Men and women's condom beliefs provide an understanding of how
they use them and an approach to communicate with them to promote
more effective use (see Table 11.3). Condom use has been associated
with more positive condom attitudes (Boyd & Wandersman, 1991;
Jemmott & Jemmott, 1990; Maticka-Tyndale, 1991; Orr & Langefeld,
1993; Valdiserri et al., 1989). Intentions to use and actual condom use
have been associated with more specific beliefs of perceived susceptibility (Goodman & Cohall, 1989; Tanfer et al., 1993; Orr & Langefeld,
1993) and perceived condom benefits and barriers (DiClemente et al.,
1992; Leland & Barth, 1992; Maticka-Tyndale, 1991; Strader & Beaman,
1989; Tanfer & Rosenbaum, 1986; Tanfer et al., 1993; Walter et al., 1993).
Condom use has also been associated with perceived self-efficacy or
confidence in the ability to use condoms (Basen-Engquist & Parcel,
1992; Jemmott & Jemmott, 1992; Joffe & Radius, 1993; Kasen, Vaughan
& Walter, 1992; Walter et al., 1993).

Providers and their clients may discuss perceived condom benefits
and barriers (see Chapter 3). Once perceived barriers have been identified, ways to manage perceived condom barriers could be explored.
For example, if the client perceives that condoms interrupt sex, the
potential of having the woman put on the condom as part of foreplay
could be discussed.

Providers may work with men on improving their skills in correct
condom use. Skills as well as confidence in skills (self-efficacy) can be
improved through practicing those skills (Bandura, 1992). For example,
clients may practice correctly putting condoms on an anatomical model
while in the clinic. Men may practice correctly putting on condoms on
themselves while they are in the privacy of their homes and not within
a sexual encounter. Strategies that included the practice of putting on
condoms increased self-efficacy and intentions to use condoms (Jemmott
& Jemmott, 1992).

Providers may work with men and women on improving their abilities to communicate with their partners about condoms. As well as
practicing a skill, watching the skill of another influences self-efficacy
and skill (Bandura, 1992). For example, clients may watch a video and
then practice a skill that they viewed such as finding ways to convince
a resistant partner to use condoms. This approach is supported in
findings from research. Watching others and practicing behaviors such
as resisting social pressure and negotiating interpersonal situations
decreased unprotected sex (Kirby et al., 1991) and decreased incidence

TABLE 11.3. Condom Perceptions

Perceived Benefits of Using Condoms

Effectiveness oriented	Related to obtaining and using	Relationship oriented
Prevents pregnancy	Easy to use	Shows concern and care
Protects from STDs/HIV	Convenient	Partners appreciate
Effective	Clean	Makes male responsible
Reliable	Safe	Requires self-control of partner
	Neatness	Popular with peers
	Increases pleasure	Man is sexier
	Have sex on spur of moment	
	Putting on is a turn on	

Perceived Barriers to Using Condoms

	Related to obtaining and using	Relationship oriented
	Not enough lubrication	Partner disagrees on use
	Inconvenient	Think having sex with others
	Difficult to obtain or buy	Women with condoms are looking for sex
	Uncomfortable	Means you don't trust partner
	Slip off, break, or leak	Girls won't want to use
	Hard to get rid of after sex	Embarrassing to talk to partner
	Embarrassing	Men don't like
	Messy	Feel dirty if man wanted to use
	Ejaculate before condom on	Use with those not close to
	Unavailable (sex not planned)	Only need with prostitutes
	Interrupts sex	Men who use are jerks
	Decreases pleasure	
	Decreases romance	
	Makes sex last longer	
	Unreliable	

Sources: Beaman & Strader (1989); Brown (1984); DiClemente et al. (1992); Eldridge, Laurence, Little, Shelby, & Brasfield (1995); Forrest, Austin, Valdes, Fuentes, & Wilson (1993); Grady et al. (1993); Hingson et al (1990); Jemmott & Jemmott (1990); Kegeles et al. (1989); Keller et al (1991); Leland & Barth (1992); Maticka-Tyndale (1991); Norris & Ford (1994); Pleck, Sonenstein, & Ku (1990, 1993); Tanfer & Rosenbaum (1986); and Valdiserri, Arena, Proctor, & Bonati (1989).

of STDs (Cohen et al., 1992). Practicing communication related to sex and contraception has been reported to positively influence communication skills (Kelly et al., 1989; Solomon & DeJong, 1989), intentions to use condoms (Jemmott & Jemmott, 1992) and contraception (Kelly et al., 1989; Solomon & DeJong, 1989).

Negotiating with partners may be especially relevant for women. Men traditionally have had greater power in male–female relationships and condom use often is dependent on men's consent and initiative (Liskin et al., 1990). Discussion with women about their right to refuse sex if their partner declines condom use is suggested (Libbus, 1992). Caution is advocated as a woman client in an abusive relationship may put herself at greater risk when asking for condom use.

EVALUATION

Condoms may be evaluated for effectiveness in relation to consistent and correct use and problems with use. Questions that may be asked to evaluate effectiveness of use include:

- How often do you have sex?
- How often do you use condoms?
- How and when do you put on the condom?
- How and when do you remove the condom?
- What if any lubrication do you use?
- What concerns do you have about using condoms?
- Have you had any negative experiences with using condoms?
- What were those negative experiences?

The ultimate evaluation is for effectiveness in preventing pregnancies and STDs. This effectiveness is related to correct and consistent use. In addition, it is important to evaluate problems experienced which may impact consistent and correct condom use. Re-education and counseling may address incorrect and inconsistent use as well as identified problems.

Effectiveness may be related to condom breakage and slippage. Condom breakage and slippage occur in a relatively few couples (Steiner et al., 1993) and may be related to sexual behavior. Condom failures have been associated with minimal foreplay and lubrication (Albert, Hatcher, & Graves, 1991) and more vigorous sex (Consumer Reports, 1989; Steiner et al., 1993). Extra-strong condoms with additional lubrication (Steiner et al., 1993) or spermicides for extra lubrication (Kestelman & Trussell, 1991) may be recommended.

Breakage and slippage may be related to incorrect condom use which may be due to insufficient experience and information. Condom breakage and slippage has been associated with less condom experience among women (Vessey et al., 1988) and couples (Steiner et al., 1993). Insufficient experience and information may lead to incorrect use such as unrolling prior to putting it on, putting it on with the rim on the inside of the condom, fingernail snags, genital contact prior to putting on the condom, and allowing the condom to slip off (Lisken et al., 1990). Other failures may be associated with incorrect care of condoms such as poor storage and the use of oil-based lubricants (Lisken et al., 1990). Latex condoms are weakened when exposed to light, heat, humidity (Lisken et al., 1990), and oil-based lubricants (Voeller et al., 1989).

Inconsistent condom use may be related to problems. Examples of problems include discomfort, breakage or slippage, unplanned sex, lack of lubrication, and interruption of sex (Forrest et al., 1993; Keller, 1993; Norris & Ford, 1993; Ross, 1987). Buying and carrying condoms prior to any potential sexual encounter could be discussed to address nonuse when sex was not planned. Condom choices may be discussed to address uncomfortableness or poor fit. The Hugger by Ansell is smaller and the Trojan Enz Larger or Magnum by Carter are larger than standard size (Billow, 1992). For slippage concerns, the Mentor by Carter, which has an adhesive that attaches to the base of the penis, may be recommended (Billow, 1992).

Another problem may be an allergic reaction to condoms. The allergic reactions may be from latex, lubricants, or spermicides. A recommendation would be to switch to another brand to eliminate the source (Billow, 1992). A solution to latex allergy would be to use both a latex and natural condom (Billow, 1992). A natural is worn over a latex condom if the woman is allergic while a latex is worn over a natural condom if the man is allergic (Billow, 1992). Another possibility is using the new polyurethane condom.

SUMMARY

Promotion of condom use is suggested based upon assessment and evaluation information. Past condom use, health risks, potential benefits, and side effects need to be assessed. The information can be used in providing education, in collaborating and in facilitating skills. Finally, evaluation needs to address consistent and correct condom use, problems and health risks.

REFERENCES

Albert, A., Hatcher, R., & Graves, W. (1991). Condom use and breakage among women in a municipal hospital family planning clinic. *Contraception, 43,* 167–176.

Bandura, A. (1992). A social cognitive approach to the exercise of control over AIDS infection. In R. DiClemente (Ed.), *Adolescents and AIDS: A generation in jeopardy* (pp. 89–116). Newbury Park: SAGE.

Basen-Engquist, K., & Parcel, G. S. (1992). Attitudes, norms, and self-efficacy: A model of adolescents' HIV-related sexual risk behavior. *Health Education Quarterly, 19,* 263–277.

Beaman, M., & Strader, M. (1989). STD patients' knowledge about AIDS and attitudes toward condom use. *Journal of Community Health Nursing, 6,* 155–164.

Billows, J. A. (1992). Choosing condoms. *American Pharmacy, NS32*(9), 55–58.

Bird, K. (1991). The use of spermicide containing nonoxynol-9 in the prevention of HIV infection. *AIDS, 5,* 791–796.

Boyd, B., & Wandersman, A. (1991). Predicting undergraduate condom use with the Fishbein and Ajzen and the Triandis attitude-behavior models. *Journal of Applied Social Psychology, 21,* 1810–1830.

Brown, I. (1984). Development of a scale to measure attitude toward the condom as a method of birth control. *The Journal of Sex Research, 20,* 255–263.

Can you rely on condoms? (March, 1989). *Consumer Reports,* pp. 135–141.

Catania, J., Coates, T., Kegeles, S., Fullilove, M., Peterson, J., Marin, B., Siegel, D., & Hulley, S. (1992). Condom use in multi-ethnic neighborhoods of San Francisco: The population-based AMEN (AIDS in multi-ethnic neighborhoods) study. *American Journal of Public Health, 82,* 284–287.

Cates, W., & Stone, K. (1992). Family planning, sexually transmitted diseases and contraceptive choice: A literature update—Part I. *Family Planning Perspectives, 24,* 75–84.

Center for Disease Control. (1992). Condom use among male injecting-drug users—New York City, 1987–1990. *Mortality & Morbidity Weekly Report, 41*(34), 617–620.

Center for Disease Control. (1993). Distribution of STD clinic patients along a stage-of-behavioral-change continuum—selected sites, 1993. *Mortality & Morbidity Weekly Report, 42*(45), 880–883.

Center for Disease Control. (1994). Health Risk behaviors among adolescents who do and do not attend school—United States, 1992. *Mortality & Morbidity Weekly Report, 43*(8), 129–132.

Cohen, D., MacKinnon, D., Dent, C., Mason, H., & Sullivan, E. (1992). Group counseling at STD clinics to promote use of condoms. *Public Health Reports, 107,* 727–731.

Contraceptive Technology Update. (1995a). FDA: Polyurethane condom carries "extremely misleading" label. *Contraceptive Technology Update, 16,* 17–22.

Contraceptive Technology Update. (1995b). Barriers to better condom "killing people"; regulatory, political hurdles stifle development. *Contraceptive Technology Update, 16,* 1–9.

DiClemente, R., Durbin, M., Siegel, D., Krasnovsky, F., Lazarus, N., & Comacho, T. (1992). Determinants of condom use among junior high school students in a minority, inner-city school district. *Pediatrics, 89,* 197–202.

Eldridge, G., Laurence, J., Little, C., Shelby, M., & Brasfield, T. (1995). Barriers to condom use and barrier method preferences among low-income African-American women. *Women and Health, 23,* 73–89.

Forrest, J., & Fordyce, R. (1993). Women's contraceptive attitudes and use in 1992. *Family Planning Perspectives, 25,* 175–179.

Forrest, K., Austin, D., Valdes, M., Fuentes, E., & Wilson, S. (1993). Exploring norms and beliefs related to AIDS prevention among California Hispanic men. *Family Planning Perspectives, 25,* 111–117.

Galavotti, C., & Schnell, D. (1994). Relationship between contraceptive method choice and beliefs about HIV and pregnancy prevention. *Sexually Transmitted Diseases, 21,* 5–7.

Goodman, E., & Cohall, A. (1989). Acquired immunodeficiency syndrome and adolescents: Knowledge, attitudes, beliefs, and behaviors in a New York City adolescent minority population. *Pediatrics, 84,* 36–42.

Grady, W., Klepinger, D., Billy, J., & Tanfer, K. (1993). Condom characteristics: The perception and preferences of men in the United States. *Family Planning Perspectives, 25,* 67–73.

Hatcher, R., Trussell, J., Stewart, F., Stewart, G., Kowal, D., Guest, F., Cates, W., & Policar, M. (1994). *Contraceptive Technology.* New York: Irvington Publishers.

Hingson, R., Strunin, L., Berlin, B., & Heeren, T. (1990). Beliefs about AIDS, use of alcohol and drugs, and unprotected sex among Massachusetts adolescents. *American Journal of Public Health, 80,* 295–299.

Jemmott, J., & Jemmott, L. (1993). Alcohol and drug use during sexual activity: Predicting HIV-risk related behaviors of inner-city black male adolescents. *Journal of Adolescent Research, 8,* 41–57.

Jemmott, L., & Jemmott, J. (1990). Sexual knowledge, attitudes, and risky sexual behavior among inner-city black male adolescents. *Journal of Adolescent Research, 5,* 346–369.

Jemmott, L., & Jemmott, J. (1992). Increasing condom-use intentions among sexually active black adolescent women. *Nursing Research, 41,* 273–279.

Joffe, A., & Radius, S. (1993). Self-efficacy and intent to use condoms among entering college freshman. *Journal of Adolescent Health, 14,* 262–268.

Jones, E., & Forrest, J. (1992). Contraceptive failure rates based on the 1988 NSFG. *Family Planning Perspectives, 24,* 12–19.

Kasen S., Vaughan, R., & Walter, H. (1992). Self-efficacy for AIDS preventive behaviors among tenth grade students. *Health Education Quarterly, 19,* 187–202.

Kegeles, S., Adler, N., & Irwin, C. (1989). Adolescents and condoms. *American Journal of Disease of Children, 143,* 911–915.

Keller, M. (1993). Why don't young adults protect themselves against sexual transmission of HIV? Possible answers to a complex question. *AIDS Education and Prevention, 5,* 220–233.

Keller, S., Bartlett, J., Schleifer, S., Johnson, R., Pinner, E., & Delaney, B. (1991). HIV-relevant sexual behavior among a healthy inner-city heterosexual adolescent population in an endemic area of HIV. *Journal of Adolescent Health, 12,* 44–48.

Kelly, J., Lawrence, J., Hood, H., & Brasfield, T. (1989). Behavioral intervention to reduce AIDS risk activities. *Journal of Consulting and Clinical Psychology, 57,* 60–67.

Kestelman, P., & Trussell, J. (1991). Efficacy of the simultaneous use of condoms and spermicides. *Family Planning Perspectives, 23,* 226–227.

Kirby, D., Barth, R., Leland, N., & Fetro, J. (1991). Reducing the risk: Impact of a new curriculum on sexual risk-taking. *Family Planning Perspectives, 23,* 253–263.

Kost, K., & Forrest, J. (1992). American women's sexual behavior and exposure to risk of sexually transmitted diseases. *Family Planning Perspectives, 24,* 244–254.

Leland, N., & Barth, R. (1992). Gender differences in knowledge, intentions, and behaviors concerning pregnancy and sexually transmitted disease prevention among adolescents. *Journal of Adolescent Health, 13,* 589–599.

Libbus, M. (1992). Condoms as primary prevention in sexually active women. *American Journal of Maternal Child Nursing, 17,* 256–260.

Lisken, L., Wharton, C., & Blackburn, R. (1990). Condoms—Now more than ever. *Population Reports, 18*(3), 1–36.

Maticka-Tyndale, E. (1991). Sexual scripts and AIDS prevention: Variations in adherence to safer-sex guidelines by heterosexual adolescents. *Journal of Sex Research, 28,* 45–66.

Mosher, W. (1990). Contraceptive practice in the United States, 1982–1988. *Family Planning Perspectives, 22,* 198–205.

Norris, A., & Ford, K. (1993). Urban, low income, African-American and Hispanic youths' negative experiences with condoms. *Nurse Practitioner, 18,* 40–48.

Norris, A., & Ford, K. (1994). Condom beliefs in urban, low income, African American and Hispanic youth. *Health Education Quarterly, 21,* 39–53.

Orr, D., & Langefeld, C. (1993). Factors associated with condom use by sexually active male adolescents at risk for sexually transmitted disease. *Pediatrics, 91,* 873–879.

Pleck, J., Sonenstein, F., & Ku, L. (1990). Contraceptive attitudes and intention to use condoms in sexually experienced and inexperienced adolescent males. *Journal of Family Issues, 11,* 294–312.

Pleck, J., Sonenstein, F., & Ku, L. (1993). Changes in adolescent males' use of and attitudes toward condoms, 1988–1991. *Family Planning Perspectives, 25,* 106–109, 117.

Ross, M. (1987). Problems associated with condom use in homosexual men. *American Journal of Public Health, 77,* 877.

Solomon, M., & DeJong, W. (1989). Preventing AIDS and other STDs through condom promotion: A patient education intervention. *American Journal of Public Health, 79,* 453–458.

Steiner, M., Piedrahita, C., Glover, L., & Joanis, C. (1993). Can condom users likely to experience condom failure be identified? *Family Planning Perspectives, 25,* 220–226.

Strader, M., & Beaman, M. (1989). College students' knowledge about AIDS and attitudes toward condom use. *Public Health Nursing, 6,* 62–66.

Tanfer, K., Grady, W., Klepinger, D., & Billy, J. (1993). Condom use among U.S. men, 1991. *Family Planning Perspectives, 25,* 61–66.

Tanfer, K., & Rosenbaum, E. (1986). Contraceptive perceptions and method choice among young single women in the United States. *Studies in Family Planning, 17,* 269–277.

Trussell, J., & Kost, K. (1987). Contraceptive failure in the United States: A critical review of the literature. *Studies in Family Planning, 18,* 237–283.

Valdiserri, R., Arena, V., Proctor, D., & Bonati, F. (1989). The relationship between women's attitudes about condoms and their use: Implications for condom promotion programs. *American Journal of Public Health, 79,* 499–501.

Vessey, M., Villard-Mackintosh, L., McPherson, K., & Yeates, D. (1988). Factors influencing use-effectiveness of the condom. *The British Journal of Family Planning, 14,* 40–43.

Vinson, R., & Epperly, T. (1991). Counseling patients on proper use of condoms. *American Family Physician, 43,* 2081–2085.

Voeller, B., Coulson, A., Bernstein, G., & Nakamura, R. (1989). Mineral oil lubricants cause rapid deterioration of latex condoms. *Contraception, 39,* 95–102.

Walter, H., Vaughan, R., Gladis, M., Ragin, D., Kasen, S., & Cohall, A. (1993). Factors associated with AIDS-related behavioral intentions among high school students in an AIDS epicenter. *Health Education Quarterly, 20,* 409–420.

CHAPTER TWELVE

Natural Family Planning and Fertility Awareness

Dona J. Lethbridge

Natural family planning (NFP), which may also be termed fertility awareness, may well be the fertility management method that most relates sexual activity to reproduction. During any episode of sexual intercourse, there is a greater or lesser likelihood that an ovum will be traveling through the fallopian tubes and able to be fertilized. This method of fertility management depends on the calculation of when ovulation is taking place and when the ovum is capable of being fertilized. It is the premise of this book that every woman should know the time of the month when she is most likely to be fertile, unless she is using hormonal birth control or sterilization, where fertility is not an issue. In an ideal relationship, a woman's partner would also know where she was in her menstrual cycle at any time.

Teachers and serious practitioners of natural family planning differentiate it from fertility awareness, however, in that natural family planning presumes sexual abstinence during the time of the menstrual month considered fertile, if pregnancy is to be avoided. Those who practice fertility awareness, knowing they are likely to be fertile on certain days, use a barrier method of contraception or a sexual behavior that does not include vaginal intercourse at those times. Natural family planning is supported by the Roman Catholic Church, as consistent with its teaching on family planning. It may also be used to plan pregnancy, since the days that pregnancy is most likely to occur are also known.

It is not known how many women use variations of natural family planning as their contraceptive method. The National Survey of Family Growth (N.S.F.G.) classified methods involving the calculation of infertile days as "periodic abstinence" and shows only 1.4% of women using the method, including natural family planning (Mosher & Pratt, 1990). However, in this survey, contraceptive use is classified by the most effective method in use. Thus, those women having unprotected intercourse on perceived infertile days would be classified only by the method (usually barrier) used during the rest of the cycle. Use of fertility awareness may vary from careful use of natural or symptothermal family planning to casual calculation of menstrual cycle dates. Since it is not an approved contraceptive method by many health care providers, women may be reluctant to admit to its use.

A study was made of women's interest in learning NFP, where women were mailed a description of the sympto-thermal method and then questioned by telephone about the potential that they would adopt the method (Stanford, Lemaire, & Fox, 1994). Of this group of middle-class women, 43% were interested in learning more, 24% said they were likely to use NFP to avoid pregnancy, and 32% were likely to use NFP to achieve pregnancy.

During in-depth interviews of their experience with contraception, women admitted calculating days of infertility or "safe days" as a contraceptive strategy in itself or as a way to make the use of barrier methods more tolerable (Lethbridge, 1991). During midcycle, women abstained from sexual intercourse or used barrier methods during the days they considered themselves fertile. Women's descriptions of their use of infertile days violates the assumption underlying contraceptive research and counseling practices, that a contraceptive method must be used during any episode of intercourse. For instance, Helbig (1987) in a study of 1,298 women attending family planning clinics, used the term contraceptive risk-taking to describe episodes of unprotected intercourse. The most distinguishing factor was the women's estimate of subjective probability of pregnancy, or estimate that they would become pregnant during an episode of unprotected intercourse. In other words, women calculated infertile days, which was termed contraceptive risk-taking.

Women may miscalculate or be unaware of mistimed ovulation and become pregnant. Miller (1975) studied women with unwanted pregnancies and described their belief that they were in the safe days of the month when they became pregnant as rationalizations for unprotected intercourse—"retrospective rhythm." Luker (1975) also described the subjective probability of pregnancy and suggested that women discounted the probability if they engaged in successful contraceptive risk-taking over time. Further study is needed of women's use of infertile days as a contraceptive strategy, especially those women who have used this method successfully.

EFFECTIVENESS OF NFP AND FERTILITY AWARENESS

A meta-analysis was performed by Kambic (1991) on 23 studies to determine the effectiveness of various methods of NFP. The use effectiveness rate ranged from 2.5 to 27.9. The use effectiveness of later studies was better than earlier ones, probably because of better teaching techniques and resources available.

In a study of the Creighton model, characterized by an introductory session, follow-up teaching sessions, evaluations, and a rigorous teacher training program (Hilgers et al., 1992), the method related effectiveness was 0 at 1 month, .4 at the 6th month, 1.2 at 12 months—where the method was perceived to have been used correctly, but a pregnancy occurred (Fehring, Lawrence, & Philpot, 1994). The Creighton model does not calculate user-related failures in the same way as is done with other methods. In this model, if a couple know they are fertile through their calculations and have genital contact anyway, they are considered to have had an achieving-related pregnancy; that is, the method was used to achieve a pregnancy and was successful. Thus, there is no consideration given to the couple who lacked the strength to resist desire.

USE OF THE COMPONENTS OF NATURAL FAMILY PLANNING

Signs of pending fertility are assessment of cervical mucus (used exclusively with the Billings Method, and with formalized, standardized training and observations in the Creighton model); the sympto-thermal method, which combines the assessment of cervical mucus with measurement of basal body temperature, and additional symptoms of ovulation, such as cervical position, mittelschmerz, postovulatory breast tenderness; daily basal body temperatures alone; or the calendar rhythm method. It is generally advised that women or couples be taught NFP by a trained and accredited educator. However, many women do not have access to or the resources for an educational program. Indeed, the World Health Organization (1981) successfully taught 869 women in 5 third-world countries, by lay trainers, using cervical mucus observation to interpret their fertility. Thus, it is conceivable that nurses and other health professionals could teach fertility awareness to all their clients of childbearing potential.

Guidelines for teaching components of NFP and fertility awareness may include the following*:

- Cervical Mucus Observation. For external observation, consider how the vagina feels first thing upon awakening or when first urinating. If the cervical mucus is dry or pasty and crumbly, the vaginal area will feel dry. Creamy or stretchy mucus will be felt on the vaginal opening and seen on the toilet paper. Feel the mucus with the fingers—If the fingers are drawn apart, is it stretchy, or does it just form little peaks? Does it feel pasty, crumbly, sticky, stretchy, and slippery? Check it often throughout the day. Learn to be conscious of how the vagina feels, whether wet or dry, without having to check.

For internal observation, this may be done at the same time as checking the position and consistency of the cervix. Wash the hands and then insert one or two fingers into the vagina. How high does the cervix feel? Is it firm like the tip of a nose or softer like the lips of a mouth? Does the cervical opening feel closed or open like a small hole? With two fingers, gently squeeze the cervix and feel the cervical mucus from the opening. Check the mucus as above.

- Basal Body Temperature Observation. The BBT thermometer is marked in one-tenths of degrees, and the markings are generally more easily read than a fever thermometer. They tend to cost about $12 at drugstores. A fever thermometer is marked in two-tenths of degrees and, if a BBT thermometer is not available, could be used.

Take the temperature as soon as you awaken, before getting out of bed or engaging in any activity, about the same time every day. Take it orally, rectally, or vaginally for 5 minutes, and in the same place every morning for consistency (a provider should show the woman how to properly use the thermometer). A rectal or vaginal temperature is about 1 full degree higher than an oral temperature. Record the temperature. Note anything unusual that may have affected the temperature, such as taking a drink, awakening later or earlier than usual, sleeping poorly, or feeling ill. If the mercury is between two lines, the lower one is recorded.

---

*Note: An excellent, very readable teaching text written for the lay person is: *The Fertility Awareness Handbook* by Barbara Kass-Annese, RN, CNP and Hal Danzer, MD, San Bernadino, CA: Borgo Press, 1992.

LEARNING THE PATTERN OF
CHECKING FERTILITY SIGNS

Once you become accustomed to checking your temperature and cervix, it will become routine. Once you know you have passed your fertile period for the month, you may stop checking the cervix and BBT until after the next menstrual cycle begins.

Therefore, each of the components of fertility awareness will be described below.

CERVICAL MUCUS OBSERVATIONS

Cervical mucus is produced by cryptlike cells lining the endocervix. It is secreted at the rate of 20 to 60 milligrams per day, except during the time around ovulation, during which it is increased tenfold (Hilgers, 1978). It changes over the course of the menstrual cycle through the influence of estrogen and progesterone, and may enhance or discourage passage of sperm through the cervix. Type E (estrogen-stimulated) mucus appears approximately 6 days before ovulation and is clear, stretchy, and lubricative. Microscopically, it is characterized by channels in its structure that facilitate the passage of sperm. Type G (progesterone-stimulated) mucus appears after ovulation and is thick, opaque, and sticky. Microscopically, the channels have become crossed and closed so that the passage of sperm is prohibited.

When learning NFP, women are taught to recognize the characteristics of their cervical mucus and its relation to their menstrual cycle. At the beginning of the menstrual cycle, as menstrual bleeding is ceasing, there may be no cervical mucus. These are called "dry days," and may be accompanied by a feeling of dryness in the tissue surrounding the vagina. As development of the follicle begins, and estrogen is released, cervical mucus will develop that is sticky, pasty, or crumbly, and looks like library paste. As ovulation approaches, the cervical mucus becomes wetter, so that this pasty mucus evolves into a creamy white mucus. This mucus will evolve into a thinner, stretchy mucus with the texture of egg white. This is called Spinnbarkeit, German for spider web. This stretchy mucus shows that ovulation has taken place or is impending. As progesterone levels rise after ovulation, the cervical mucus becomes sticky, pasty, and dry. It may feel that way for the rest of the cycle or change to a thinner, wetter, though still-infertile mucus, before the next menses begins.

Since sperm may live only a few hours without type E mucus and up to 5 days with type E mucus, and the ovum is presumed to last 6 to 24 hours after ovulation, the fertile period is presumed to start with the first sign of Spinnbarkeit, and continue until a day of dry, sticky mucus has occurred. Proponents of formal, religiously based NFP emphasize periods of abstinence. Within this form of NFP, sexual abstinence would begin at the first sign of Spinnbarkeit, and continue throughout the presumed fertile period. Sexual abstinence is also considered necessary on every second day throughout the follicular phase of the menstrual cycle, when cervical mucus is being observed. This is so that post-coital semen does not mask cervical mucus.

Those using a nonreligiously based NFP, fertility awareness, may use another form of birth control during the fertile days or sexual behavior that does not include vaginal penetration. During the follicular phase, when it is necessary to carefully observe mucus, rather than abstinence, couples may limit intercourse to evenings, and void immediately afterwards to enable semen to escape rather than pool and remain in the vagina. It may also be useful to examine mucus obtained from the tip of the cervix, that is, that most recently released, if intercourse has recently occurred, to decrease confusion with remaining semen.

BASAL BODY TEMPERATURE

Basal body temperature (BBT) is the temperature of the body at rest, best assessed just upon awakening, before any daily activity. The BBT is measured with a finely graded thermometer, enabling observation of changes of tenths of a degree from day to day. The principle behind the use of BBT in reflecting ovulation is that the presence of progesterone raises the temperature. Thus, at the beginning of the menstrual cycle, the temperature may be somewhat raised from the progesterone of the previous cycle, but will soon drop and remain low. Shortly before, during, or after ovulation, the BBT will rise to a higher level, from 3/10 (.3) of a degree to 1 degree higher than previously. It will stay at a higher level throughout the rest of that cycle, beginning to fall as menses begin. If it stays high longer than 20 days, and intercourse took place midcycle, it may be a sign of pregnancy. Because it is not certain at exactly what point around ovulation the temperature rises, it is not considered an adequate sign of when the fertile period is occurring. In many cases, it will be indicating that ovulation has already occurred. However, when used in conjunction with cervical mucus observation, it can help to pinpoint the day of ovulation. Monthly calendars that aid in charting BBT and other signs of fertility are available in the packaging of BBT thermometers as well as from health care providers through various drug representatives.

CERVICAL POSITION

Another sign of the fertile stage is the position and consistency of the cervix. During menses, the cervix is low in the vagina and the os is open to permit menstrual flow. As menses end and the menstrual cycle ensues, the cervix will be low with the os closed, and will feel like the cartilage at the tip of the nose. A nulliparous woman will feel the os as small and circular, a parous woman as wider and irregularly shaped. As ovulation approaches, the cervix rises in the vagina, softens, and the os opens. It has been described as feeling more like lips at this stage rather than the tip of the nose. This higher position helps the sperm to travel into the os of the cervix. After ovulation, the rising progesterone level causes the cervix to lower and become firmer, the os once again closed. If there is any prolapse of the uterus, as a woman has aged and borne children, it will be difficult to feel cervical position changes.

OTHER POSSIBLE SIGNS OF OVULATION

Mittelschmerz, or pain at the time of ovulation, is felt by some women. As the ovum is released with a rush of follicular fluid, slight bleeding will take place from the center of the follicle. This may leak into the pouch of Douglas in the abdominal cavity behind the vaginal posterior fornix causing mittelschmerz. There may also be some slight vaginal bloody spotting at midcycle.

There are other signs women experience after ovulation has taken place, mostly due to progesterone levels. Many women experience breast tenderness, signaling to them they are in the luteal, infertile phase of their cycle. Other luteal signs include oily skin and acne, fluid retention, mood changes, increased libido midcycle, and as menses near, abdominal cramps and backache. These are not considered reliable signs by serious users of NFP that ovulation has occurred, but many women use these bodily changes as indications of their ovulatory status.

Recently, findings from a study of menstrual cycles, hormonal fluctuations, and the occurrences of conceptions suggest that fertilization may only occur from 6 days before until the day of ovulation (Wilcox, Weinberg, & Baird, 1995). This is especially startling because it suggests that unless the ovum is fertilized upon release from the ovary, it is nonfertile thereafter. If this is the case, the key may be sperm available in the woman's reproductive tract from intercourse preceding ovulation, and that sperm may be present and able to fertilize the ova for up to 6 days. This would make natural family planning even more difficult to use, since accurate prediction of ovulation, using cervical mucus and BBT, is more likely as the time of release of the ova nears. Yet the woman may be most fertile during this period. If these new findings are supported, natural family planning guidelines will have to be amended, so that vaginal intercourse is avoided during much of the follicular stage. Couples will be also be able to be more confident that pregnancy is not possible once the luteal phase is apparent.

SPECIAL CIRCUMSTANCES

ILLNESS AND FEVER

A fever will mask BBT changes. If a fever occurs, the woman should switch to a normal thermometer, since the BBT thermometer just goes up to 99 degrees Fahrenheit. In addition, an illness could delay the follicular stage, causing ovulation to occur late, or prohibit ovulation from occurring, with cyclical bleeding occurring or not. Cervical mucus patterns may continue to be observed during an illness. If ovulation does occur, even if late, type E mucus should be observed. If the cycle is anovulatory, there may be sticky, pasty mucus throughout; there may be no mucus and the vagina may remain dry; wet, creamy mucus may occur but not evolve into Spinnbarkeit.

If a vaginal infection occurs, cervical mucus can be masked. Vaginal discharge may differ from cervical mucus in that it may have an odor, be yellow, or in the case of candida albicans, be white and pasty, but accompanied by redness and itching. Vaginal creams and suppository treatments will also mask cervical mucus. In these cases the woman will have to rely on BBT, and generally abstain from intercourse until the infection clears up.

BREAST-FEEDING

While a woman is completely breast-feeding an infant, without any supplemental feeding, ovulation may be delayed. When a woman has had a number of children, and totally breast-fed them, she may have experienced the return of menses around the same time after each birth. The challenge for most women, however, is knowing when ovulation has returned and the woman is once again fertile (Lethbridge, 1989).* As the infant grows, and spaces between breast-feedings widen, there may be sporadic follicle ripening and estrogen release. Thus, cervical mucus sporadically may seem to be signaling the onset of ovulation, but it may continue to be delayed. Cervical mucus may be dry, alternate with pasty days and dry days, occasional creamy days, and as ovulation nears, a more normal pattern of pasty to creamy to sticky mucus. The woman should be observing her cervical position during this time as an additional sign of her ovulatory status. Ovulation may return if breast-feeding becomes sporadic, such as when a mother returns to work, or if the infant begins to sleep through the night. Some serious practitioners of NFP suggest actively encouraging the return of ovulation through giving the infant supplemental feedings, so that the couple may return to a predictable ovulatory pattern (Richards, 1978).

If a postpartum woman does not breast-feed, she can ovulate as soon as 2 weeks after delivery. It is difficult to check cervical mucus when she is still passing lochia, but as soon as lochia ceases she should return to her prepregnancy NFP observations.

THE PERIMENOPAUSAL PERIOD

Once again, sporadic follicle ripening may be occurring, resulting in prolonged menstrual cycles, with delayed ovulation and menses, or anovulatory cycles with cyclical bleeding or no bleeding. Menstrual cycles may shorten considerably, possibly averaging 20 to 26 days, as the perimenopausal period begins. Even if ovulation occurs, if the follicular stage is 9 days or less, the released ovum is probably immature, and the cycle is considered anovulatory (Metcalfe, 1979). As the perimenopausal period continues, cycles will lengthen with follicles possibly ripening, but not sufficiently to release enough estrogen to decrease FSH and stimulate the LH surge and ovum release. During a long anovulatory stage, cervical mucus may either be dry or be in a constant state, whether pasty or white and creamy. After a year without menses, the chances of ovulation occurring are decreased greatly, though a conservative rule is to wait for 2 years before assuming cessation of ovulation if a woman is under 50.

---

*From Lethbridge, D. J. (1989). The use of breastfeeding as a contraceptive. *Journal of Obstetric, Gynecologic and Neonatal Nursing, 18,* 31–37. Copyright © 1989 by Lippincott-Raven. Adapted with permission.

STRATEGIES FOR INTERVENTION

Two issues are important. Do the woman and man wish to use natural family planning in its most formal sense because of religious or moral reasons, or are they more oriented to learning fertility awareness to more effectively use contraception? Additionally, it is generally recommended that couples learn these techniques through formal teaching programs. In fact, the Creighton method includes a formal teaching program as one of its essential components. Not all women and couples, however, have access to teaching programs, either because of availability or resources. Following is a list of resources available to those interested in natural family planning.

American Academy of Natural Family Planning
11700 Stuet Avenue
St. Louis, MO 63141
(314) 991-5766

Billings Ovulation Method Association
8514 Bradmoor Drive
Bethesda, MD 20817
(301) 897-9323

The Couple to Couple League International, Inc.
PO Box 11084
Cincinnati, OH 45211
(513) 661-7612

Northwest Family Services
4805 N.E. Glisan
Portland, OR 97213
(503) 230-6377

Pope Paul VI Institute for the Study of Human Reproduction
6901 Mercy Road
Omaha, NE 68106
(402) 390-6600

In reality, a resourceful health care provider may teach women and men the components of natural family planning or fertility awareness. In fact, fertility awareness, where all women, and ideally their partner, had the means to know the days when they were most likely to be fertile, would be an excellent enhancement to a family planning teaching plan. The limited contraceptive options available to women and men necessitate providing all resources possible, including knowledge of their own bodily functioning.

REFERENCES

Fehring, R. J., Lawrence, D., & Philpot, C. (1994). Use effectiveness of the Creighton Model Ovulation Method of natural family planning. *Journal of Obstetrical, Gynecologic and Neonatal Nursing, 23,* 303–309.

Helbig, D. (1987). *Components of effective fertility regulation.* (Report No. R01-HD-16504). Washington, D.C.: National Institute of Child Health Development, Center for Population Research.

Hilgers, T. (1978). Cervical mucus. In Fr. A. Zimmerman (Ed.), *A reader in natural family planning.* Collegeville, MN: The Human Life Center, pp. 38–39.

Hilgers, T. W., Daly, K. D., Prebil, A. M., & Hilgers, S. K. (1992). Cumulative pregnancy rates in patients with apparently normal fertility and fertility-focused intercourse. *Journal of Reproductive Medicine, 37,* 864–866.

Kambic, R. T. (1991). Natural family planning use-effectiveness and continuation. *American Journal of Obstetrics and Gynecology, 165*(Suppl.), 2046–2048.

Kass-Annese, B., & Danzer, H. (1992). *The fertility awareness handbook.* San Bernadino, CA: Borgo Press.

Lethbridge, D. J. (1989). The use of breastfeeding as a contraceptive. *Journal of Obstetrical, Gynecologic and Neonatal Nursing, 18,* 31–37.

Lethbridge, D. J. (1991). Women's experience with contraception: Towards a theory of contraceptive self-care. *Nursing Research, 40,* 276–280.

Luker, K. (1975). *Taking chances: Abortion and the decision not to contracept.* Berkeley, CA: University of California Press.

Metcalfe, M. (1979). Incidence of ovulatory cycles in women approaching the menopause. *Journal of Biosocial Science, 11*(1), 39–48.

Miller, W. B. (1975). Psychological antecedents to conception among abortion seekers. *Western Journal of Medicine, 122,* 12–19.

Mosher, W. D., & Pratt, W. F. (1990). Contraceptive use in the United States, 1973–1988. *Advance data from vital and health statistics, No. 182.* Hyattsville, MD: National Center for Health Statistics.

Richards, F. (1978). NFP guidance during the post-partum. In Fr. A. Zimmerman (Ed.), *A reader in natural family planning.* Collegeville, MN: The Human Life Center, 33–37.

Stanfield, J. B., Lemaire, J. C., & Fox, A. (1994). Interest in natural family planning among female family practice patients. *Family Practice Research Journal, 14,* 237–249.

Wilcox, A. J., Weinberg, C. R., & Baird, D. D. (1995). Timing of sexual intercourse in relation to ovulation. Effects of the probability of conception, survival of the pregnancy, and sex of the baby. *New England Journal Of Medicine, 333*(23), 1517–1521.

World Health Organization. (1981). A prospective multicentre trial of the ovulation method of natural family planning. II. The effectiveness phase. *Fertility and Sterility, 36,* 591–598.

Ancient Methods of Fertility Regulation

Dona J. Lethbridge

In much of the world, methods of contraception used since early times are still in use. In western countries, probably more than family planning health care practitioners will ever know, women and men use these ancient methods as creative, generally frowned-upon, emergency methods of contraception on some, and sometimes many, occasions. A sensitive, nonjudgmental practitioner may be able to learn strategies couples use to prevent a conception after they have had relatively "unprotected" intercourse. We need to recognize that some of these methods, such as coitus interruptus, are time-honored methods of contraception, were used very often before modern methods became available. Since these methods are no longer considered acceptable by many health care providers, only rudimentary, if any, effectiveness data are available. It is possible that methods such as coitus interruptus, combined with fertility awareness, may be relatively effective, if used deliberately and diligently (Lethbridge, 1991).* In this chapter, the contraceptive use and effects of breast-feeding, coitus interruptus, and douching will be discussed.

---

*From Lethbridge, D. J. (1991). Coitus interruptus: Considerations as a method of birth control. *Journal of Obstetrical, Gynecologic and Neonatal Nursing, 20,* 80–85. Copyright © 1991 by Lippincott-Raven. Adapted with permission.

BREAST-FEEDING AS A METHOD
OF CONTRACEPTION

Breast-feeding generally is considered an unreliable method of contraception, and postpartum mothers are routinely warned by health care professionals against counting on breast-feeding to prevent another pregnancy. Yet, breast-feeding is probably nature's way of controlling births and enabling mothers to space pregnancies. Breast-feeding may be useful for mothers wanting to delay subsequent pregnancies, and who are unwilling or unable to use other birth control methods (Lethbridge, 1989).*

Evidence exists that women in developing parts of the world space their children through the use of breast-feeding. The recently nomadic Kung had a mean birth interval of 4.1 years (Konner & Worthman, 1980). In rural Rwanda women, 75% of subsequent conceptions occurred between 24 and 29 months postpartum (Bonte, Akingeneye, & Gashakamba, 1974). In Chile among exclusively breast-feeding women, only 6% were pregnant at 18 months postpartum (Zacharias et al., 1987). All of these women who exclusively breast-fed, kept their infants with them at all times, including sleeping with them. In some of these cases, infants suckle approximately every 15 to 20 minutes for brief periods throughout the day and night. Nutritional status had a small effect on delayed anovulation, but only in cases where it was very poor (Lunn et al., 1980; Menken, Trussell, & Watkins, 1981). In India, it was found that amenorrhea was delayed in breast-feeding women in those who were older, but was earlier in those of higher income and social status (Nath et al., 1993). American women, tending to be comparatively well nourished, also have very different breast-feeding patterns. Women who fully breast-feed tend to feed their infants 8 times per day for 20-minute periods and, as soon as possible, train their infants to sleep through the night. Thus, the state of amenorrhea due to breast-feeding may be considerably shorter in western women. In two studies of western women who breast-fed their infants frequently throughout the day and night and allowed the infants to wean naturally averaged 14.5 and 11.4 months, respectively before the return of menses (Kippley & Kippley, 1972; Knauer, 1985).

The principal problem with using breast-feeding as a contraceptive is that determining when ovulation has returned is difficult. Studies

---

*From Lethbridge, D. J. (1989). The use of breastfeeding as a contraceptive. *Journal of Obstetrical, Gynecologic and Neonatal Nursing, 18,* 31–37. Copyright © 1989 by Lippincott-Raven. Adapted with permission.

investigating whether ovulation occurs before the first menses suggest that menses are more apt to be anovulatory if they occur closely after the birth, or if the woman is more fully breast-feeding (Perez et al., 1972). Thus, longer breast-feeding periods may be related to ovulation predating the return of menses.

The process by which breast-feeding prevents ovulation is not fully understood. It is probable that prolactin levels discourage the release of LH by the anterior pituitary (Baird et al., 1979; Bonnar et al., 1975). Prolactin levels have been found to rise during pregnancy, to 200 mg/ml at term (Jaffe et al., 1973). Prolactin levels remain higher in breast-feeding women than in those who are partially breast-feeding and fall more rapidly to prepregnancy levels for those who do not breast-feed by the end of the third postpartum week than for those who do breast-feed by that time (Bonnar et al., 1975; Howie et al., 1981).

Prolactin is produced by the anterior pituitary under control of the hypothalamus. The role of the hypothalamus is probably inhibitory because any disruption of the pituitary-hypothalamic pathway results in hyperprolactinemia (Daniel & Prichard, 1975). The hypothalamus produces two balancing hormones: prolactin-inhibiting factor and pro-lactin-producing factor. The prolactin-inhibiting factor is thought to be closely associated with dopamine and is inhibited according to the frequency, intensity, and duration of the sucking stimulus, resulting in the secretion of prolactin.

Prolactin may change the sensitivity of the hypothalamus to increased levels of estrogen, depressing the release of LH-releasing hormone (McNeilly, 1979). High levels of prolactin may also directly affect ovarian response to LH and FSH, preventing the induction of ovulation (McNatty, Sawers, & McNeilly, 1974). Gonadotropins may have a decreased response to gonadotropin-releasing hormone during lactation (Mishell & Marrs, 1986). Women administered bromocriptine, a prolactin-inhibiting medication, were found to have a lack of gonadotropin response to gonadotropin-releasing hormone similar to that observed in lactating woman. The other possible mechanism is that through neural stimulation of the nipple through sucking, beta endorphins are released that suppress the hypothalamic gonadotropin-releasing hormone (Short, 1984). Resumed ovulatory activity was seen when amenorrhea arising from an excess of prolactin was treated with naloxone, even though prolactin levels remained high (Lamberts, Timmers, & DeJong, 1981).

Should breast-feeding continue for a prolonged period, however, prolactin levels eventually will decrease and menses will resume. Menstrual periods, and probably ovulation, may be irregular in the breast-feeding woman, depending on increased or decreased breast-feeding activity (Gross & Eastman, 1985).

If a woman desires to try to inhibit ovulation as long as possible through breast-feeding, it has been suggested that at least 5 breast-feedings per day with a total duration of more than 65 minutes is necessary, and that continuation of night breast-feeding is necessary (McNeilly et al., 1983). In a study of early versus late menstruators postpartum in breast-feeding women, early menstruators' infants slept through the night a mean of 8.6 months, versus a mean of 19.3 months for late menstruators (Knauer, 1985). "Complete breast-feeding," which may be most successful in delaying ovulation consists of the use of the breast for pacification, continued night feedings, breast-feeding according to the infant's desire, and minimal separation of mother and baby (Kipley & Kipley, 1972; 1979). After the infant begins to eat solid foods (after 6 months), complete breast-feeding continues until the infant loses interest.

In family planning programs throughout the world, the lactational amenorrhea method (LAM) has been implemented as an effective way to space births, even after the introduction of supplementary foods (Huffman & Labbok, 1994; Perez, Labbok, & Queenan, 1992; Ravera et al., 1995). Using LAM, statistics such as one woman in 422 becoming pregnant in 6 months, and pregnancy rates of 2.9 at 6 months and 5.9 at 12 months have been found (Kennedy & Visness, 1992; Perez, Labbok, & Queenan, 1992). These pregnancy rates are similar to those with other established contraceptive methods. In studies of LAM, it was found using hormone studies that if breast-feeding continued unabated and frequently, there would be continued amenorrhea (Gross, 1991).

Identifying the woman for whom breast-feeding is a viable and appropriate contraceptive method is important. Because other methods of birth control, such as barrier methods, are safe to use during breast-feeding, provide effective protection against pregnancy, and do not rely on the necessary determination of the onset of ovulation, these methods are probably superior. The woman using breast-feeding as a contraceptive must be either highly motivated to avoid another pregnancy or planning on another pregnancy spaced by breast-feeding activity (Labbok et al., 1991). The postponement of ovulation requires diligence in breast-feeding activity and attention to bodily changes that indicate the onset of ovulation (see Chapter 12 on Natural Family Planning and Fertility Awareness). The cooperation of the partner is essential for the woman to undertake complete breast-feeding involving the constant presence of the infant and maintenance of night feedings.

The mother's work plans are also important, since unless she is able to have the infant with her at home or at the workplace, sufficient breast-feeding to maintain an anovulatory state is probably difficult. Though milk expression may be used to maintain lactation, the nipple stimulation of suckling is necessary to maintain prolactin levels, and it is not known if mechanical pumps provide the appropriate stimulation. She should also be referred to organizations and lactation consultants that can advise her in maintaining complete breast-feeding.

Organizations helpful to those using complete breast-feeding to delay ovulation include:

International Childbirth Education Association
P. O. Box 20852
Milwaukee, WI 53220
(414) 476-0130

International Lactation Consultant Organization
P. O. Box 4031
University of Virginia Station
Charlottesville, VA 22903
(708) 328-7385

La Leche League International
9616 Minneapolis Avenue
Franklin Park, IL 60131
(312) 455-7730

COITUS INTERRUPTUS (WITHDRAWAL)

Coitus interruptus has probably been used throughout history, and continues to be used today, to space and prevent births (Lethbridge, 1991).* Coitus interruptus is referred to somewhat negatively in the Bible and the Talmud, and more positively in the ninth century writings of Islamic prophets. It was probably used widely during the Middle Ages to prevent births, since fewer than expected mean family sizes have been found in British ducal families in the 14th century, in European ruling families, and villages in the 18th century.

---

*From Lethbridge, D. J. (1991). Coitus interruptus: Considerations as a method of birth control. *Journal of Obstetrical, Gynecologic and Neonatal Nursing, 20,* 80–85. Copyright © 1991 by Lippincott-Raven. Adapted with permission.

Coitus interruptus is used today as a method of birth control. In 1982, the World Fertility Survey indicated that 30% of women in Belgium reported its use for family planning. Similarly, 44% of women in Spain, 29% in France, and 23% in Hungary reported use of this method. One article suggests that coitus interruptus is, in fact, an acceptable, and even respectable, method of contraception because its successful use has connotations of restraint (Schneider & Schneider, 1991).

The use of coitus interruptus is reportedly far less in the United States, but the practice continues by those who perceive that they have no other available methods. For example, in a study of 625 young urban African American males, aged 11 to 19, 87% were sexually active, and almost 40% did not use any form of birth control during their most recent act of intercourse. Of those who did, 56% used a male method (i.e., condoms or withdrawal) and almost 15% used withdrawal. In 1976, in a national study on the sexual experiences of adolescents, 17.2% who had used contraceptives stated that coitus interruptus was the first method they ever used. In addition 16.9% had used coitus interruptus as the method of birth control in their most recent sexual encounter. Similarly, in a national study of premarital sexual intercourse, 23.7% of female respondents reported coitus interruptus was used during their first episode of sexual intercourse.

The NSFG study reports that fewer than 2% of females aged 15 to 44 use coitus interruptus. This population represents females from all socioeconomic groups and stages of childbearing. However, in a study of women of upper socioeconomic class, almost 9% used coitus interruptus at least some of the time, and the use of it and the rhythm method increased with the greater number of previous contraceptive methods used (Lethbridge, 1990). This finding is similar to another study of women undergoing tubal sterilization. Women who had used more past methods of contraception had switched to either the rhythm method or coitus interruptus before undergoing sterilization. Study results seem to indicate that, in the United States, two types of individuals are more likely to use coitus interruptus: those who do not perceive the availability of other contraceptive methods, and those who have exhausted all other available methods.

Findings regarding the effectiveness of coitus interruptus are mixed. In 1961, Westoff et al. listed the failure rate as 15.6% (that is, in one year, approximately 16 of 100 women would become pregnant). Recent data have not been available on the effectiveness of coitus interruptus, either in the general population or among specific groups of users. Past users, of course, may have been more practiced in the method. Perceived effectiveness in preventing a pregnancy is a prime consideration in an individual's choice of a contraceptive method. Therefore, women and men faced with a situation of unprotected intercourse may choose coitus interruptus as the only method available, thinking it better than no method at all.

PHYSIOLOGIC CONSIDERATIONS

Generally, coitus interruptus is considered ineffective in preventing pregnancy, most frequently because of the belief that pre-ejaculatory fluid contains sperm. This idea stems from the writings of Stone, who reported in 1931 the testing of 24 samples of pre-ejaculatory fluid collected from 18 men. He found that two samples showed many spermatozoa, two contained a few, one had an occasional sperm. The remaining 19 samples showed no spermatozoa. How Stone defined pre-ejaculatory fluid and how he collected the fluid from his subjects are unknown. Some of the samples may have contained actual ejaculatory fluid. Subsequent studies of the sperm contact of pre-ejaculatory fluid have not been reported.

Masters and Johnson measured pre-ejaculatory fluid. They described it as mucoid in character and consisting of usually no more than two or three drops of fluid. It is more likely to occur during long maintained, plateau-phase sexual tension levels. It is believed to originate in the urethral glands, such as Cowper's gland.

It is quite possible that failures of this method of birth control are not due to pre-ejaculatory fluid. Generally, at least 10 million spermatozoa per milliliter (a number generally considered to be below the normal level of spermatozoa) are necessary to fertilize an ovum. The vas deferens and cauda epididymidis together contain 70% of the mature spermatozoa with fertilizing ability and motility. The vas deferens contains only 2%. Therefore, even in a case of a higher than normal sperm count, such as 250 million per milliliter, a pre-ejaculatory emission containing sperm from the vas deferens would contain only 5 million spermatozoa. This emission also would lack the ejaculatory force necessary to propel sperm through the female reproductive tract.

Failure of coitus interruptus most probably occurs because of a couple's inability to use the method effectively and regularly. The man requires self-control to withdraw the penis just before orgasm. Not only must he be highly motivated and disciplined to comply, but he must be able to accurately predict when his orgasm will occur. This may be especially difficult for men in their teens and early 20s, who have a stronger sexual drive than older men, and for whom the onset of orgasm may be rapid and unpredictable. Also, at the time of orgasm, many men maintain deep, unmoving vaginal penetration when seminal emission occurs. For these men, withdrawal at the time of orgasm would be an unnatural and unpleasant event.

The use of coitus interruptus also may be unsatisfactory for women. A woman may feel sexually frustrated if the man withdraws during coitus. In some cases, male orgasm results in the cessation of coitus because penile detumescence occurs soon after orgasm. If, during coitus, the woman is mutually orgasmic with her partner, his withdrawal would be especially unpleasant.

TEACHING AND COUNSELING IMPLICATIONS

Many questions remain about coitus interruptus that can only be answered with empirical data. Nevertheless, coitus interruptus is a method of contraception used by some couples, and may serve as an alternative for those with no other method at a time when they will not forgo sexual intercourse.

Health care practitioners may have ethical difficulty teaching about coitus interruptus as a contraceptive technique, tantamount to condoning the use of a theoretically less effective method, as well as a method that does not protect against sexually transmitted disease. Since coitus interruptus is generally described as ineffective, counselors may give the message, and even believe, that using coitus interruptus is no better than using no method at all when existing knowledge about theoretical effectiveness rates suggest this to be untrue. Health care practitioners must be willing and able to give full information about birth control methods so that women and men can make informed decisions about the best method available to them.

DOUCHING

In the United States, there are no data as to how much douching is used as a contraceptive method, regularly or occasionally. Since the N.S.F.G. denotes the method used as the most effective when more than one method is indicated, douching will probably go unnoted in almost all cases. In the Soviet Union, where there is a shortage of contraceptive methods, 13% of women use douching as their sole method (Visser et al., 1993). In Nigeria, soft drinks as douches are included as available vaginal chemical contraceptives in an area where few resources are available for contraception (Nwoha, 1992).

Vaginal douching is probably practiced regularly by 20 million American women. In an early study of American women in military sites in Germany, over half of the women practiced douching on a regular basis (Stock, Stock, & Hutto, 1973). In another early study, douching was so accepted as a contraceptive technique that college girls' knowledge of the method was tested in a study of contraceptive information (Grinder & Schmitt, 1966). In a recent study of 618 women seeking gynecological care, 59% had douched at some time, 12% douched at least once a month, and 3% at least once a week (Rosenberg, Phillips, & Holmes, 1991). Those who practiced douching were more likely to be African American, less educated and younger, and to have a lower family income. They were less likely to use spermicides or barrier contraceptives. A national marketing study cited in Rosenberg, Phillips, and Holms (1991), suggests that of the U.S. population of 92 million women, 73% (67 million) have douched at some time, 37% (34 million) had douched within the last 6 months, and 24% (22 million) had douched within the previous month. African American women were far more likely to use douching.

In a study of 142 adolescents in a family planning clinic in Texas, 69% reported douching, with 81% of the African American respondents, 48% of the Hispanics, and 46% of the Anglos (Chacko et al., 1989). Twenty percent reported douching once a week, 25% twice a week, and 6% more than 3 times a week. Reasons given included to feel clean (67%), to prevent an odor (12%), to feel clean after a period (10%), to prevent an infection (7%), to feel clean after sex (3%), and to prevent pregnancy (1%). In another study of adolescents, with 75 boys and 88 girls in rural New York state, 21% of those who were sexually active relied on the contraceptive methods of withdrawal and douching (McCormick, Izzo, & Folcik, 1985). Use of these methods was related to a low frequency of sexual intercourse, and teens reported also relying on "luck" because of their infrequent exposure to pregnancy.

The question remains as to how well douching after intercourse might work as a spermicide. Commercial douche instructions state that douching will not prevent conception or cure or prevent a vaginal infection. Indeed, it is suggested that 5 minutes after ejaculation, sperm have reached the fallopian tubes. During the fertile phase of the menstrual cycle, sperm are also stored in the channels formed in the cervical mucus for later release during subsequent hours. Are these initial numbers of sperm adequate to fertilize a waiting ovum? Will douching rid the vagina of the rest of the spermatozoa pooled in the vagina and in the cervical mucus? In a study of the persistence of spermatozoa in the lower genital tracts of 675 women at varying times after intercourse, of those who had douched after coitus, 48% still had spermatozoa in cervico-vaginal smears within 2 days of coitus (Silverman & Silverman, 1978). However, the number of live spermatozoa was very small.

It stands to reason that douching may provide some protection against pregnancy. When couples with problems of infertility are pursuing pregnancy, the woman is instructed to have intercourse in the supine position to maintain the ejaculate in the vaginal pool. She is also instructed to stay reclining for at least one half hour after intercourse. If a woman selects the superior position in intercourse, and then stands up and douches within 5 minutes, might she not greatly reduce the number of spermatozoa available for fertilization? In a study in Nigeria, where douching is an accepted method of contraception, common douching solutions were tested for their spermicidal properties (Nwoha, 1992)). They tested three cola drinks available in Nigeria, including Coca Cola, and Krest bitter lemon, another drink commonly used for douching. While the cola drinks had mixed success as spermicides, all leaving some live sperm, the bitter lemon was completely successful in killing all sperm within one minute.

It is not the purpose of this chapter to recommend douching as a contraceptive technique, but to acknowledge its use by some, especially those with few other resources. It is clear that douching is used by many women for hygienic reasons and this may mask post-coital use as a contraceptive. There is increased literature suggesting that douching leads to an increased risk of vaginal infections and ascending infections, including pelvic inflammatory disease, but these are still inconclusive (Grodstein & Rothman, 1994; Jossens, Schachter, & Sweet, 1994; Rosenberg & Phillips, 1992; Spinillo et al., 1993). It is not clear whether douching causes organisms to move through the cervix into the higher reproductive tract, or whether douching is used by those with a higher risk of infections and as a self-treatment.

Douching with hydrostatic pressure probably does increase the risk of infection and should be strongly discouraged. During pregnancy, douching may increase the risk of uterine embolism, a potentially fatal syndrome, and should also be discouraged for that reason. Women should be taught that the vagina has a natural cleansing action because of its acidic environment, and that douching may in fact interfere with this.

REFERENCES

Atighetchi, D. (1994). The position of Islamic tradition on contraception. *Medical Law, 13*(4), 717–725.

Baird, D. T., McNeilly, A. S., Sawers, R. S., & Sharpe, R. M. (1979). Failure of estrogen-induced discharge of luteinizing hormone in lactating women. *Journal of Clinical and Endocrinological Metabolism, 49,* 500–506.

Bonnar, J., Franklin, M., Nott, P. N., & McNeilly, A. S. (1975). Effect of breastfeeding on pituitary-ovarian function after childbirth. *British Medical Journal, 4,* 82–84.

Bonte, M., Akingeneye, E., Gashakamba, M., Mbarutso, E., & Nolens, M. (1974). Influence of the socioeconomic level on the conception rate during lactation. *International Journal of Fertility, 19,* 97–102.

Chacko, M. R., McGill, L., Johnson, T. C., Smith, P. G., & Nenney, S. W. (1989). Vaginal douching in teenagers attending a family planning clinic. *Journal of Adolescent Health Care, 10,* 217–219.

Clark, S. D., Zabin, L. S., & Hardy, J. B. (1984). Sex, contraception and parenthood: Experience and attitudes among urban black young men. *Family Planning Perspectives, 16,* 77–82.

Creatsas, G. K. (1993). Sexuality: Sexual activity and contraception during adolescence. *Current Opinion in Obstetrics and Gynecology, 5*(6), 774–783.

Daniel, P. M., & Prichard, M. M. L. (1975). Studies of the hypothalamus and pituitary gland. *Acta Endocrinologa, 80,* 201–207.

Grinder, R. E., & Schmitt, S. S. (1966). Coeds and contraceptive information. *Journal of Marriage and the Family, 28,* 471–479.

Grodstein, F., & Rothman, K. J. (1994). Epidemiology of pelvic inflammatory disease. *Epidemiology, 5*(2), 234–242.

Gross, B. A. (1991). Is the lactational amenorrhea method a part of natural family planning? Biology and policy. *Obstetrics and Gynecology, 165*(6, pt. 2), 2014–2019.

Gross, B. A., & Eastman, C. J. (1985). Prolactin and the return of ovulation in breast-feeding women. *Journal of Biosocial Science, 9*(Suppl.), 25–42.

Howie, P. W., McNeilly, A. S., Houston, M. J., Cook, A., & Boyle, H. (1981). Effect of supplementary food suckling patterns and ovarian activity during lactation. *British Medical Journal, 283,* 757–759.

Huffman, S. L., & Labbok, M. H. (1994). Breastfeeding in family planning programs: A help or a hindrance? *International Journal of Gynecology and Obstetrics, 47*(Suppl.), S23–S31.

Jaffe, R. B., Yuen, B. H., Keye, W. R., & Midgley, A. R. (1973). Physiologic and pathologic profiles of circulating human prolactin. *American Journal of Obstetrics and Gynecology, 117,* 757–773.

Jossens, M. O., Schachter, J., & Sweet, R. L. (1994). Risk factors associated with pelvic inflammatory disease of differing microbial etiologies. *Obstetrics and Gynecology, 83*(6), 989–997.

Kennedy, K. I., & Visness, C. M. (1992). Contraceptive efficacy of lactational amenorrhoea. *Lancet, 339*(8787), 227–230.

Kippley, J. F., & Kippley, S. K. (1972). The relation between breastfeeding and amenorrhea. *Journal of Obstetrical, Gynecologic and Neonatal Nursing, 1*(4), 15–21.

Kippley, J. F., & Kippley, S. K. (1979). *The art of natural family planning.* Cincinnati, Ohio: The Couple to Couple League.

Knauer, M. (1985). Breastfeeding and the return of menstruation in urban Canadian mothers practicing "natural mothering." In V. Hull & M. Simpson (Eds.), *Child health, and child spacing: Cross-cultural perspectives* (pp. 187–211). Dover, NH: Croom Helm.

Konner, M., & Worthman, C. (1980). Nursing frequency, gonadal function and birth spacing among Kung hunter-gatherers. *Science, 207,* 788–792.

Labbok, M. H., Stallings, R. Y., Shah, F., Perez, A., Klaus, H., Jacobson, M., & Maruthi, T. (1991). Ovulation method use during breastfeeding: Is there increased risk of unplanned pregnancy? *American Journal of Obstetrics and Gynecology, 165*(6, Pt. 2), 2031–2036.

Lamberts, S. W. J., Timmers, J. M., & DeJong, F. H. (1981). The effect of long-term naloxone infusion on the response of gonadotropins to luteinizing hormone-releasing hormone and on plasma estradiol concentration in a patient with a prolactin-secreting pituitary adenoma. *Fertility and Sterility, 36,* 678–681.

Lethbridge, D. J. (1989). The use of breastfeeding as a contraceptive. *Journal of Obstetrical, Gynecologic and Neonatal Nursing, 18,* 31–37.

Lethbridge, D. J. (1990). The contraceptive use of women of upper socio-economic status. *Health Care for Women International, 11,* 305–318.

Lethbridge, D. J. (1991). Coitus interruptus: Considerations as a method of birth control. *Journal of Obstetrical, Gynecologic and Neonatal Nursing, 20,* 80–85.

Lunn, P. G., Prentice, A. M., Austin, S., & Whitehead, R. G. (1980). Influence of maternal diet on plasma-prolactin levels during lactation. *Lancet, 1,* 623–625.

McCormick, N., Izzo, A., & Folcik, J. (1985). Adolescents' values, sexuality, and contraception in a rural New York county. *Adolescence, 20,* 385–395.

McNeilly, A. S. (1979). Effects of lactation on fertility. *British Medical Bulletin, 35,* 151–154.

McNeilly, A. S., Glasier, A. F., Howie, P. W., Houston, M. J., Cook, A. , & Boyle, H. (1983). Fertility after childbirth: Pregnancy associated with breast feeding. *Clinical Endocrinology, 18,* 167–173.

McNatty, K. P., Sawers, R. S., & McNeilly, A. S. (1974). A possible role for prolactin in control of steroid secretion in the human graafian follicle. *Nature, 250*(5468), 653–655.

Menken, J., Trussell, J., & Watkins, S. (1981). The nutrition fertility link: An evaluation of the evidence. *Journal of Interdisciplinary History, 11,* 434–437.

Mishell, D. R. & Marrs, R. P. (1986). Endocrinology of lactation and the puerperium. In D. R. Mishell & V. Davajan (Eds.), *Infertility, contraception and reproductive endocrinology.* Oradell, NJ: Medical Economics Books.

Nwoha, P. U. (1992). The immobilization of all spermatozoa in vitro by bitter lemon drink and the effect of alkaline pH. *Contraception, 46,* 537–542.

Nath, D. C., Singh, K. K., Land, K. C., & Talukdar, P. K. (1993). Breastfeeding and postpartum amenorrhea in a traditional society: A hazards model analysis. *Social Biology, 40*(1-2), 74–86.

Perez, A., Labbok, M. H., & Queenan, J. T. (1992). Clinical study of the lactational amenorrhoea method for family planning. *Lancet, 339*(8799), 968–970.

Perez, A., Vela, P., Masnick, G. S., & Potter, R. G. (1972). First ovulation after childbirth: The effect of breastfeeding. *American Journal of Obstetrics and Gynecology, 114,* 1041–1047.

Ravera, M., Ravera, C., Reggiori, A., Cocozza, E., Cianta, F., Riccioni, G., & Kleimayr, R. (1995). A study of breastfeeding and the return of menses in Hoima District, Uganda. *East African Medical Journal, 72*(3), 147–149.

Rogow, D., & Horowitz, S. (1995). Withdrawal: A review of the literature and an agenda for research. *Studies in Family Planning, 26*(3), 140–153.

Rosenberg, M. J., & Phillips, R. S. (1992). Does douching promote ascending infection? *Journal of Reproductive Medicine, 37,* 930–938.

Rosenberg, M. J., Phillips, R. S., & Holmes, M. D. (1991). Vaginal douching: Who and why? *Journal of Reproductive Medicine, 36,* 753–758.

Scheider, J., & Schneider, P. (1991). Sex and respectability in an age of fertility decline: A Sicilian case study. *Social Science Medicine, 33*(8), 885–895.

Short, R. V. (1984). Breast feeding. *Scientific American, 250*(4), 35–41.

Silverman, E. M., & Silverman, A. G. (1978). Persistence of spermatozoa in the lower genital tracts of women. *Journal of the American Medical Association, 240,* 1875–1877.

Spinollo, A., Pizzoli, G., Colonna, L., Nicola, S., De Seta, F., & Guaschino, S. (1993). Epidemiologic characteristics of women with idiopathic recurrent vulvovaginal candidiasis. *Obstetrics and Gynecology, 81*(5, Pt. 1), 721–727.

Stock, R. J., Stock, M. E., & Hutto, J. M. (1973). Vaginal douching: Current concepts and practices. *Obstetrics and Gynecology, 42,* 141–146.

Tay, C. C. (1991). Mechanisms controlling lactational infertility. *Journal of Human Lactation, 7*(1), 15–18.

Taylor, H. W., Smith, R. E., & Samuels, S. J. (1991). Post-partum anovulation in nursing mothers. *Journal of Tropical Pediatrics, 37*(6), 286–292.

Visser, A. P., Pavlenko, I., Remmenick, L., Bruyniks, N., & Lehert, P. (1993). Contraceptive practice and attitudes in former Soviet women. *Advances in Contraception, 9,* 13–23.

Zacharias, S., Aguilera, E., Assenzo, J., & Zanartu, J. (1987). Return of fertility in lactating and nonlactating women. *Journal of Biosocial Science, 19,* 163–169.

The IUD

Dona J. Lethbridge

The Intrauterine Device (IUD) is a small plastic or metal apparatus inserted into the uterus to prevent pregnancy. It is thought to be an ancient method of contraception, with reports that in early times, small stones were placed in the uteri of camels to prevent conception during estrus. While the IUD is infrequently used in the United States, it is much more commonly used in other parts of the world. In addition, new methods are under development that combine the use of the device with a hormone-releasing mechanism that may lead to its increased use in the future.

The IUD has been in disregard and was unavailable in the United States for several years. A large case control study was conducted in the late 1970s examining the association between IUD use and the risk of pelvic inflammatory disease (PID) requiring hospitalization (Burkman and the Women's Health Study, 1981; Lee et al., 1983). The article by Burkman and colleagues estimated the risk of PID to be 1.6 for IUD users and 2.1 for those who had no history of previous STDs. They did not separate out a risk for the Dalkon Shield. The study by Lee and colleagues estimated a risk of 1.6 for PID among IUD users with no history of PID and 8.3 among Dalkon Shield users. These findings were published at the time of the litigation against the A. H. Robbins company who manufactured the Dalkon Shield, and who later filed for bankruptcy protection. Other makers of IUDs discontinued production, fearing similar lawsuits. Since that period, the Women's Health Study data, considered most influential on the fate of the IUD, has been critiqued for sources of bias (Petitti, 1992). From using PID cases that had been hospitalized, to including women with a history of PID in the sample group, to the difficulty of diagnosing PID, to the use of data collectors who were not blind about groups member of subjects, it was suggested that the risk of PID might have been substantially exaggerated (Kronmal, Whitney, & Mumford, 1991). The findings of Lee and colleagues (1983) of a relative risk of 1.6 for IUD use other than Dalkon Shield use is probably more accurate. At 2.0% of women who use contraception using the IUD, its use is just beginning to resume in the United States (Mosher & Pratt, 1990). Following cessation of the Dalkon Shield and the FDA's recommendation to remove IUDs in case of pregnancy, there have been no deaths reported in the United States with an IUD in situ in a 5-year period (Sivin, 1993).

MECHANISM OF ACTION

It is still not truly known how the IUD functions to prevent pregnancy. For years, it was thought that the IUD was an abortifacient. It was thought to set up an inflammatory response in the endometrium such that it was inhospitable to a fertilized ovum. This chronic endometritis has been found in most IUD users, and in one study of women who became pregnant with an IUD, only 6% were found to have endometritis (Ezra, Birkenfeld, & Levij, 1989). Anti-inflammatory agents such as aspirin have been found to be used with greater frequency in women who became pregnant with an IUD (Papiernik, Rozenbaum, Amblard, Dephot, & de Mouzon, 1989). On the other hand, high prostaglandin levels, thought to be associated with the chronic endometritis of the IUD, have not been found. In a study of uterine washings in new IUD users and experienced users, prostaglandin levels were found to be high post insertion, but low in experienced users, suggesting that the initial high levels were more likely due to post-insertion increased bleeding and pain (El-Sahwi et al., 1987).

In recent years, it is thought that the IUD acts more as a spermicide, hormone-releasing IUDs hindering sperm from penetrating cervical mucus, IUDs generally phagocytizing sperm with leukocytes, incapacitating them with head-tail separation in the presence of copper, as well as other cytotoxic effects in the IUD-altered uterine fluid. In the oviducts of copper IUD users, ova are less frequently found than in controls (Sivin, 1989). In a study of the number of blighted early pregnancies, as indicated by HCG levels, among women using an IUD, there was no transient rise of HCG in the IUD group (Segal et al., 1985). Finally, in a search made for ova in women using IUDs versus those using no contraception, during the midcycle peak of LH, ova were recovered from tubal flushings in 39% of IUD users compared to 56% of control group women (Alvarez et al., 1988). Eggs with a microscopic appearance consistent with fertilization were recovered from 50% of the control women who had intercourse during the fertile period of their cycle. No such ova were recovered from the women with IUDs who had intercourse within the fertile period. No ova were found in the body of the uterus in any of the IUD users.

It may be that IUDs operate as a combination of several mechanisms, as a spermicide and, in hormone-releasing devices, as an anti-ovulatory device, but also making the endometrium inhospitable to implantation. A description of the IUD as a successful postcoital contraceptive suggests that its insertion and subsequent endometrial changes might inhibit implantation if conception did occur (Gottardi, Spreafico, & Orchi, 1986). Thus, those women and men most concerned about the IUD being an abortifacient might be able to accept a hormone-releasing device, most likely to affect sperm effectiveness and ovulation as its dominant mechanism, if the IUD is a good choice for other reasons.

IUDS IN USE

At the time of this writing, only two IUDs are available in the United States: the Paragard T380A and the Progestasert. Another, levonorgestrel-releasing IUD has undergone clinical testing in the United States and is widely used in other countries. It may therefore eventually be approved for use in the United States.

THE PARAGARD T380

This IUD is a T-shaped device with copper on both arms and the stem, that is placed into the uterine fundus. The exposed surface areas of copper are $380 +/- 23$ mm^2. It is 36 mm along the arms and 32 mm along the stem. The product pamphlet asserts that the T380 must be replaced every 4 years, though a study of women in Hungary showed very low pregnancy rates up to 10 years after insertion, with lower loads of copper (Batar, 1992). In studies of IUDs with similar amounts of copper, there was no change in serum copper levels from before use, to 1 month and to 12 months after insertion of the devices, suggesting that copper stays localized (Arowojolu, Otolorin, & Ladipo, 1989). In studies of pregnancy rates between copper IUDs containing 380 mm^2 and 200 mm^2, 0.5 and 2.6 pregnancies per 100 women were found, respectively (Farr & Amatya, 1994). Similar results were found with 375 mm^2 and 250 mm^2 copper IUDs (Castro, Abarca, & Rios, 1993). No significantly different differences were found in expulsion or removals due to bleeding, pain, inflammations or infections, or insertion-related events. The IUD users with the higher levels of copper, however, were found to report increased dysmenorrhea.

THE PROGESTASERT (ALZA CORPORATION)

The Progestasert is a white, T-shaped IUD constructed of ethylene/vinyl acetate containing titanium dioxide, and is placed into the uterine fundus. The T-arm is 32 mm, the stem is 36 mm, and it contains a reservoir of 38 mg of progesterone. Progesterone is released at an average rate of 65 mcg per day for 1 year by membrane controlled diffusion from the reservoir. The progesterone is localized. Serum concentrations of LH, estradiol, and progesterone indicate cyclic patterns indicative of ovulation during use of the Progestasert. However, endometrial proliferation is suppressed, possibly inhibiting sperm survival, or the inability of the endometrium to form a cavity for implantation. The Progestasert must be replaced every 12 months.

LEVONORGESTREL-RELEASING IUDS (LEIRAS CORPORATION)

The levonorgestrel-releasing (LNG) IUD is T-shaped, constructed of polyethylene, with the stem lined with the active ingredient levonorgestrel. A membrane controls the release of hormone into the uterus at a constant rate of 20 mcg per day. It shows promise as having extremely low pregnancy rates and decreasing the risk of pelvic inflammatory disease (PID). Decreases in menstrual flow, however, have led to discontinuation of the device for some women. In a study of the function of this device, fewer than half of menstrual cycles examined by ultrasound showed normal follicular growth and rupture (Barbosa et al., 1990). When ovulation did occur, progesterone cycles were lower than controls. Preovulatory estradiol and LH peak levels were also lower. In another study, women using the LNG IUD were also found to have significantly higher rates of amenorrhea, delayed ovarian follicular atresia, skin and hair conditions, and headache, all possibly related to progestin effects (Sivin & Stern, 1991). Thus, unlike the Progestasert, LNG IUDs may have a systemic effect on gonadotropin secretion, which disturbs follicular development.

These hormonal changes would be an additional contraceptive effect, in addition to endometrial changes. With the use of progesterone-releasing IUDs, dilated, thin-walled vesicles, associated with a thinning of the surface epithelium, and a decidual reaction in the stroma occurred over 6 months time (Sheppard, 1987). With the LNG-IUD, a uniform suppression of the functional endometrium throughout the uterus occurred after only 4 weeks.

In a comparison of a copper-containing IUD and the LNG IUD, pregnancy rates were 5.9% versus .5% over 5 cumulative years (Andersson, Odlind, & Rybo, 1994). The LNG IUD caused reduction of menstrual blood loss and development of oligo-amenorrhea. Therefore, termination rates for prolonged menstrual flow were significantly less. However termination rate because of amenorrhea was 6.0%. Hemoglobin levels increased during use of the LNG group and decreased with the copper device. The PID rate was low in the LNG users regardless of age, but increased in the youngest women with the copper IUD.

WOMEN'S EXPERIENCE, SIDE EFFECTS, AND RISKS WITH USE OF THE IUD

PID

The most frequently considered side effect of the IUD is PID. In a study of fallopian tube specimens of nonhormonal IUD and Progestasert users, 49% of the nonhormonal IUD users had histologically detectable salpingitis, none of whom had symptoms of PID (Soderstrom, 1983). Cultures showed the inflamed tubes to be sterile, suggesting that they might be more susceptible to infection, but were not necessarily infected. None of the Progestasert users showed any detectable salpingitis.

It is important to note, however, that PID may be symptomless and difficult to diagnose. In a study of fallopian tubes removed during tubal sterilization, of 25 women who had used the IUD in the past, 11 had evidence of inflammation compared to 2 women in the 25-women control group (Ghosh, Gupta, & Gupta, 1989). The inflammation identified was both acute and chronic, though none of the women had clinical signs.

In a comparison of copper-bearing IUDs in 937 women and LNG IUDs in 1,821 women, the cumulative 36-month gross rate of PID was 2.0 in the copper IUD and .5 in the LNG IUD (Toivonen, Luukkainen, & Allonen, 1991).

In a study of ectopic pregnancies, suggested to be secondary to the presence of PID, IUD users had a relative risk of 3.8 compared to oral contraceptive users and 3.6 compared to barrier method users (Rossing, Daling, Voigt, Stergachis, & Weiss, 1993). Women who had used an IUD in the past for 3 or more years also had a relative risk of 2.5 of ectopic pregnancy compared to those women who had never used an IUD (Rossing et al., 1993).

Those women generally at highest risk for PID are young, not married, have or have had STDs, as well as having been young at the time of first intercourse, have a high frequency of intercourse, and a large number of sexual partners (Grodstein & Rothman, 1994). The use of barrier methods or hormonal contraception decreases the risk of PID. With the use of an IUD, the risk of PID is highest shortly after insertion and in those women also at risk for STDs.

In a study with regard to insertion factors using the WHO clinical trial data of 22,908 IUD insertions and 51,299 woman-years of follow-up, and after adjustment for confounding factors, the risk for PID was more than six times higher during the 20 days after insertion than during later times (Farley et al., 1992). Further, the risk was low and constant for up to 8 years of follow-up—1.6 cases per 1,000 woman-years of use.

IUD strings have also been tested as possible vectors for PID organisms, but evidence suggests that it does not play an important role. In a study of 1,265 women, randomly assigned to receive a standard copper bearing IUD that does not normally have a significantly discernible string, and a version of the device with a marker string, no difference was found in the incidence of PID or other types of infection or inflammation (Potts et al., 1991).

RETURN OF FERTILITY AFTER IUD USE

In a study of the return of fertility after IUD use, however, perhaps one of the most important factors in the risk of PID, in 91 women who discontinued various types of IUD because of desired pregnancy, the pregnancy rates at 3, 6, 12, and 18 months after removal were 61.5, 87.9, 92.3, and 96.7%, respectively (Gupta, Gupta, & Lyall, 1989). The mean interval to conception after removal of the IUD was 4.4 months. In another study, examining only copper-bearing IUD use, 79.3% of women were pregnant after 11 months and 90.4 after 23 months observation (Skjeldestad & Bratt, 1987). There were no significant differences in the type of IUD, duration of use, or maternal age. However, parous women showed a tendency to become pregnant more readily than nulliparous women.

CHANGES IN MENSTRUAL PATTERNS

Discontinuation of the IUD seems to be related mostly to physiological factors such as menstrual changes and pain, and this occurs most frequently with nulliparous women. IUDs such as the Lippes Loop and copper-bearing IUDs have long been known to increase the length and amount of menstrual flow.

In a study of iron status in women 35 to 65 years, s-ferritin levels were most dependent on length of menstrual bleeding, which was related to method of contraception and lowest in premenopausal women who used the IUD (Milman et al., 1993). S-ferritin values representing small and depleted iron stores were found in 61% of IUD users. In a test of menstrual blood loss with the Lippes Loop, copper-bearing IUDs and the Progestasert, blood loss was greatest with the Lippes Loop (Andrade et al., 1988). There was increased blood loss of 1 to 17 ml of menstrual blood in the first 6 months after insertion, returning to pre-insertion levels after 6 months. Serum ferritin levels were lower for 1 year and then returned to admission values. Progestasert users had a reduction of 40 to 50% in menstrual blood loss and an increase in serum ferritin. In more in-depth study, this research team estimated normal menstrual blood loss at about 32 ml per month (Andrade, Pizarro, & Orchard, 1987). This increased to 52–72 ml with nonmedicated IUDs and this did not change over 24 months time. Lower levels of copper on IUDs increased blood loss to 37–40 ml the first month and decreased to 30–38 ml after 1 year of use. Higher copper levels' blood loss was 56–63 ml at first, evening out to 45–73 ml at 2 years. Progestogen-releasing IUD's mean blood loss was 27–36 ml at 1 month and 9–13 ml at 12 months. Intermenstrual blood loss was significant only in the first month post-insertion.

On the other hand, with the LNG IUD, the change in bleeding pattern was the most frequent reason for discontinuation, with removal for amenorrhea cited (Wang et al., 1992). The percentage of women with amenorrhea was 29.3% at the end of 2 years of use. However, in a population of women with iron deficiency anemia, all IUDs lowered an already low hematocrit and ferritin levels except the LNG IUD, with which only 2% of users had a subnormal hematocrit after 41 months of use (Faundes et al., 1988).

THE OCCURRENCE OF PREGNANCY

In a test of the LNG IUD and a 380 mm² copper-containing IUD, cumulative pregnancy rates were 1.1 per 100 at 7 years for the LNG and 1.4 per 100 for the copper-releasing IUD (Sivin et al., 1991). In a study comparing an IUD in use in years past, the Lippes Loop, and a version bearing copper, accidental pregnancy rates after 1 year of use were .56 for the copper-bearing versus 4.63 for the standard Lippes Loop (Randic et al.,

1991). After 2, 4, and 10 years, these rates were 1.24, 2.70, and 3.62 versus 6.03, 7.58, and 14.94, respectively. Similarly, expulsion/displacement rates were 4.49, 4.49, 5.23, and 6.32 for the copper-bearing and 12.61, 13.29, 15.46, and 19.79 for the standard, over periods of 1, 2, 4, and 10 years. Thus, it appears that the use of copper has made a marked difference in the effectiveness of the IUD. The LNG IUD also seems to have an extremely low failure rate. With all methods, though, nulliparous women are at greatest risk for an accidental pregnancy (Bracher & Santow, 1992).

ENDOMETRIAL CANCER

In a large, multi-center, population-based case-control study in the United States, 437 women 20 to 54 years old with epithelial endometrial carcinoma were compared to 3,200 controls, past IUD use was found to be strongly protective (odds ratio = .29, 95% confidence interval of .15 to .6) (Castellsaque, Thompson, & Dubrow, 1993). It was suggested that the IUD exerted a protective effect through local structural and biochemical changes in the endometrium that may alter endometrial sensitivity and response to circulating estrogen and progesterone.

STRATEGIES FOR INTERVENTION

Now that IUDs are available, federal regulations require an informed decision brochure to be read, explained, with each section initialed. Sections of the consent form include introductory material about the risks, including the possibility of death and ineffectiveness of medical treatment; effectiveness rates compared to other contraceptive methods, continuation rates, lack of contraceptive effect after removal, special risk factors, side effects, what should be discussed with the physician, adverse reactions, warnings, how it is inserted and removed, directions for use, and a special warning about uterine pregnancy with an IUD in place. Both patient and physician must then sign the document.

Though a woman has had a thorough explanation and signed a document, complete understanding of the material cannot be assumed. The language of the document is complex, and its purpose is for protection of the physician as well as informed consent. Before the woman leaves the clinic, her understanding should be evaluated and any section reviewed as needed. She should also be encouraged to keep the form for future reference. The FDA form may also provide the basis for a clinic publication oriented to the specific environment and population.

Since the expulsion rate of an IUD is highest when it is inserted postpartum (7–15 per 100 users), women must be taught to detect expulsions and instructed to return to their health care provider for reinsertion or for another method (O'Hanley & Huber, 1992). If the IUD is inserted with high fundal placement, expulsion rate will be reduced, but expert and proper insertion cannot be assumed in all cases. Those IUDs with marker strings can be checked if the woman is willing to insert her finger into her vagina to feel the presence of the string. Those with only the small filament for removal must feel the os of the cervix to ascertain the continuing presence of the IUD.

Since the rate of infection is highest in the first 20 days after insertion, this suggests that IUDs should be left in place up to their maximum lifespan and should not routinely be removed earlier, if the woman wishes to continue with the device. It also suggests that prophylactic antibiotics after insertion are a good strategy. Of course, women must be carefully counseled as to whether the IUD is the best choice for them. Those with multiple partners and a history of STDs or PID should be counseled to avoid this method and those with early onset of intercourse should have their current lifestyle assessed regarding stability of their relationship. Teaching of the symptoms of PID is necessary, including mild to significant abdominal pain or cramping, vaginal discharge, an ongoing low-grade temperature or a fever in an acute bout, and in extreme cases, severe general malaise. The need for immediate health care should be emphasized in these situations.

A most important aspect of health care is helping women to cope with the menstrual changes associated with the IUD. All devices will have some pain and bleeding after insertion. Copper-bearing devices will quite likely lead to increased flow and cramping that might last from 6 months to a year. In many cases this will even out to pre-insertion levels. In women with pre-insertion heavy menstrual flow, the use of these IUDs must be considered in light of an increase which might be unacceptable in terms of blood loss and difficult to tolerate generally. Hormone-bearing devices, on the other hand, will lead to decreased menstrual flow and in the case of the LNG-IUD to amenorrhea after about 1 year. This may be very difficult for women to understand and tolerate, and their feelings and beliefs about the role of menses in their own assessment of their health must be respected. While information that the cessation of menses is harmless should be given, amenorrhea may be intolerable for some women, and in these cases the device should be removed, with another device or contraceptive method used instead.

The increased bleeding associated with nonmedicated IUDs and the copper-bearing devices makes them unacceptable for women with marginal or severe anemia. If a woman with iron deficiency is currently using such a device and satisfied with it, iron supplements and dietary counselling are important. Hormone-bearing devices will probably be most useful for women with marginal anemia, possibly combined with teaching about the role of menstrual blood loss and loss of iron.

Finally, the IUD suffers from a poor reputation in the United States and it will take a while for this to change. One study showed that when the personal experience of peers with IUDs was shared with potential new users, they had a more favorable perspective and indicated they were most willing to try it (Cantor, Alfonso, & Zillman, 1976). In developing countries where the IUD is the predominant contraceptive used, lay workers who are also peers with personal experience are very effective in helping women become informed and accepting of this device (Fisher & de Silva, 1986). Over time, the IUD may once again become a viable contraceptive choice for women in North America, when a coital-independent method is desired.

REFERENCES

Alvarez, F., Brache, V., Fernandez, E., Guerrero, B., Guiloff, E., Hess, R., Salvatierra, A. M., & Zacharias, S. (1988). New insights on the mode of action of intrauterine contraceptive devices in women. *Fertility and Sterility, 49,* 768–773.

Andersson, K., Odlind, V., & Rybo, G. (1994). Levonorgestrel-releasing and copper-releasing (Nova-T) IUDs during five years of use: A randomized comparative trial. *Contraception, 49*(1), 56–72.

Andrade, A. T., Pizarro, E., & Orchard, E. (1987). Quantitative studies on menstrual blood loss in IUD users. *Contraception, 36,* 129–144.

Andrade, A. T., Pizarro, E., Shaw, S. T., Jr., Souza, J. P., Belsey, E. M., & Rowe, P. J. (1988). Consequences of uterine blood loss caused by various intrauterine contraceptive devices in South American women. *Contraception, 38*(1), 1–18.

Arowojolu, A. O., Otolorin, E. O., & Ladipo, O. A. (1989). Serum copper levels in users of multiload intra-uterine contraceptive devices. *African Journal of Medical Science, 18,* 295–299.

Barbosa, I., Bakos, O., Olsson, S. E., Odlind, V., & Johansson, E. D. (1990). Ovarian function during use of a levonorgestrel-releasing IUD. *Contraception, 42*(1), 51–66.

Batar, I. (1992). Clinical experiences with MLCu250 and MLCu375 IUD. *Advances in Contraception, 8*(1), 73–80.

Bracher, M., & Santow, G. (1992). Premature discontinuation of contraception in Australia. *Family Planning Perspectives, 24*(2), 58–65.

Burkman, R. T. and the Women's Health Study. (1981). Association between intrauterine device and pelvic inflammatory disease. *Obstetrics and Gynecology, 57*, 269–279.

Cantor, J. R., Alfonso, H., & Zillmann, D. (1976). The persuasive effectiveness of the peer appeal and a communicator's first-hand experience. *Communication Research, 3*, 293–310.

Castellsaque, X., Thompson, W. D., & Dubrow, R. (1993). Intra-uterine contraception and the risk of endometrial cancer. *International Journal of Cancer, 54*, 911–916.

Castro, A., Abarca, L., & Rios, M. (1993). The clinical performance of the Multiload IUD. II. The influence of age. *Advances in Contraception, 9*, 291–298.

El-Sahwi, S., Toppozada, M., Kamel, M., Gaweesh, S., Riad, W., Ibrahim, I., & el-Sabbagh, H. (1987). Prostaglandins and cellular reaction in uterine flushings. I. Effect of IUD insertion. *Advances in Contraception, 3*, 291–302.

Ezra, Y., Birkenfeld, A., & Levij, I. S. (1989). Endometrial reaction to intrauterine device in pregnancy. *Gynecologic and Obstetrical Investigation, 28*(1), 5–7.

Farley, T. M., Rosenberg, M. J., Rowe, P. J., Chen, J. H., & Meirik, O. (1992). Intrauterine devices and pelvic inflammatory disease: An international perspective. *Lancet, 339*(8796), 785–788.

Farr, G., & Amatya, R. (1994). Contraceptive efficacy of the Copper T 380A and Copper T 200 intrauterine devices: Results from a comparative clinical trial in six developing countries. *Contraception, 49*, 231–243.

Faundes, A., Alvarez, F., Brache, V., & Tejada, A. S. (1988). The role of the levonorgestrel intrauterine device in the prevention and treatment of iron deficiency anemia during fertility regulation. *International Journal of Gynecology and Obstetrics, 26*, 429–433.

Fisher, A. A., & de Silva, V. (1986). Satisfied IUD acceptors as family planning motivators in Sri Lanka. *Studies in Family Planning, 17*, 235–242.

Ghosh, K., Gupta, I., & Gupta, S. K. (1989). Asymptomatic salpingitis in intrauterine contraceptive device users. *Asia Oceania Journal of Obstetrics and Gynecology, 15*(1), 37–40.

Grodstein, F., & Rothman, K. J. (1994). Epidemiology of pelvic inflammatory disease. *Epidemiology, 5*, 234–242.

Gottardi, G., Spreafico, A., & De Orchi, L. (1986). The postcoital IUD as an effective continuing contraceptive method. *Contraception, 34,* 549–558.

Gupta, B. K., Gupta, A. N., & Lyall, S. (1989). Return of fertility in various types of IUD users. *International Journal of Fertility, 34,* 123–125.

Kronmal, R. A., Whitney, C. W., & Mumford, S. D. (1991). The intrauterine device and pelvic inflammatory disease: The Women's Health Study reanalyzed. *Journal of Clinical Epidemiology, 44,* 109–122.

Lee, N. C. et al., (1983). Type of intrauterine device and the risk of pelvic inflammatory disease. *Obstetrics and Gynecology, 62,* 1–10.

Milman, N., Rosdahl, N., Lyhne, N., Jorgensen, T., & Graudal, N. (1993). Iron status in Danish women aged 35–65 years. Relation to menstruation and method of contraception. *Acta Obstetrics and Gynecology Scandia, 72,* 601–605.

Mosher, W. D. & Pratt, W. F. (1990). Contraceptive use in the United States, 1973–1988. *Advance data from vital and health statistics; No 182.* Hyattsville, MD: National Center for Health Statistics.

O-Hanley, K., & Huber, D. H. (1992). Postpartum IUDs: Keys for success. *Contraception, 45,* 351–361.

Papiernik, E., Rozenbaum, H., Amblard, P., Dephot, N., & de Mouzon, J. (1989). Intrauterine device failure: Relation with drug use. *European Journal of Obstetrics, Gynecologic and Reproductive Biology, 32,* 205–212.

Petitti, D. B. (1992). Reconsidering the IUD. *Family Planning Perspectives, 24*(1), 33–35.

Potts, D. M., Champion, C. B., Kozuh-Novak, M., Alvarez-Sanchez, F., Santiso-Galvez, R., Tacla, X., Cohen, J., & Rivera, R. (1991). IUDs and PID: A comparative trial of strings versus stringless devices. *Advances in Contraception, 7,* 231–240.

Randic, L., Haller, H., Perovic, M., & Farr, G. (1991). The effect of adding copper onto Lippes Loop IUDs: Results from a ten-year study in Yugoslavia. *Contraception, 43,* 229–239.

Rossing, M. A., Daling, J. R., Voigt, L. F., Stergachis, A. S., & Weiss, N. S. (1993). Current use of an intrauterine device and risk of tubal pregnancy. *Epidemiology, 4,* 252–258.

Rossing, M. A., Daling, J. R., Weiss, N. S., Voigt, L. F., Stergachis, A. S., Wang, S. P., & Grayston, J. T. (1993). Past use of an intrauterine device and risk of tubal pregnancy. *Epidemiology, 4,* 245–251.

Segal, S. J., Alvarez-Sanchez, F., Adejuwon, C. A., Brache de mejia, V., Leon, P., & Faundes, A. (1985). Absence of chorionic gonadotropin in sera of women who use intrauterine devices. *Fertility and Sterility, 43,* 214–218.

Shephard, B. L. (1987). Endometrial morphological changes in IUD users: A review. *Contraception, 36*(1), 1–10.

Sivin, I. (1989). IUDs are contraceptives, nor abortifacients: A comment on research and belief. *Studies in Family Planning, 20,* 355–359.

Sivin, I. (1993). Another look at the Dalkon Shield: Meta analysis underscores its problems. *Contraception, 48*(1), 1–12.

Sivin, I., & Stern, J. (1994). Health during prolonged use of levonorgestrel 20 micrograms/d and the copper Tcu 380Ag intrauterine contraceptive devices: A multicenter study. *Fertility and Sterility, 61*(1), 70–77.

Sivin, I., Stern, J., Coutinho, E., Mattos, C. E., el Mahgoub, S., Diaz, S., Pavez, M., Alvarez, F., Brache, V., Thevenin, F., et al. (1991). Prolonged intrauterine contraception: A seven-year randomized study of the levonorgestrel 20 mcg/day (Lng 20) and the Copper T380 Ag IUDs. *Contraception, 44,* 473–480.

Skjeldestad, F. E., & Bratt, H. (1987). Return of fertility after use of IUDs (Nova-T, MLCu250 and MLCu375). *Advances in Contraception, 3,* 139–145.

Soderstrom, R. M. (1983). Will progesterone save the IUD? *Journal of Reproductive Medicine, 28,* 305–308.

Toivonen, J., Luukkainen, T., & Allonen, H. (1991). Protective effect of intrauterine release of levonorgestrel on pelvic infection: Three years' comparative experience of levenorgestrel- and copper-releasing intrauterine devices. *Obstetrics and Gynecology, 77,* 261–264.

Wang, S. L., Wu, S. C., Xin, X. M., Chen, J. H., & Gao, J. (1992). Three years' experience with levonorgestrel-releasing intrauterine device and Norplant-2 implants: A randomized comparative study. *Advances in Contraception, 8,* 105–114.

CHAPTER FIFTEEN

Tubal Sterilization and Vasectomy

Dona J. Lethbridge

S terilization has become the predominant method of contraception used in the world. The National Family Growth Study (N.S.F.G.) conducted in 1988 in the United States shows 29.7% of women between 15 and 44 are sterile through surgery or their partners' vasectomies (see Chapter 8). It has been estimated that between 600,000 and 1,000,000 women each year undergo sterilization in the United States (Bachrach et al., 1985). Sterilization is more predominantly used by African American women and women over 35. In Canada, latest statistics show 38% of women have undergone sterilization (Balakrishnan et al., 1985). The prevalence varies in other countries, ranging from minimal use in areas such as sub-Saharan Africa to 19% in Mexico, 23% in Thailand, and from 9% to 29% in the six major subregions of the Peoples Republic of China (Dwyer & Haws, 1990; Mexico National Survey on Fertility and Health, 1990; Poston, 1986; Thailand Demographic and Health Survey, 1989). Male and female sterilization procedures are considered to be relatively simple, considered permanent in spite of some possibility of reversals, and the most highly effective of contraceptive measures. This chapter will focus on sterilization procedures, men and women's responses to the actual operation, post-sterilization responses over time, and reversal procedures.

TUBAL STERILIZATION

THE PROCEDURE

Tubal sterilization is considered to be a permanent procedure that involves surgical occlusion of the fallopian tubes so that they are impassable to ova and sperm. It may be performed by division and ligation of oviducts (Pomeroy or Irving methods), most common several decades ago, and involving removing a segment of the midsection of the oviduct and folding and tying off the severed ends. In some cases, the fimbriated ends of the oviducts are removed. Electrocoagulation is occlusion by cauterization of the midsection of the oviduct. Sterilization is also carried out through the application of spring-loaded clips (Hulka, Spring or Filshie) or rings (Falope or Yoon). It is effected through laparotomy, laparoscopy, or more rarely culposcopy, and under general or local anesthesia (de Villiers & Morkel, 1987; Griffin & Mandsager, 1987; Irving, 1950; Peterson et al., 1987; WHO Task Force on Female Sterilization, 1982; Yoon & Poliakoff, 1978).

Tubal sterilization has a high success rate, in that only 1 to 2% fail to prevent pregnancy. One of the most common reasons for failure of sterilization is an early preexisting pregnancy. It is important that women be given a serum pregnancy test preoperatively. Other complications include failure because of loss or failure of fallopian rings or clips, and operative mishaps where a fallopian tube is missed and not occluded.

There has been little or no study of women's feelings about the actual operative experience of tubal sterilization. However, it may be speculated that women's relationships with health care providers may influence their perception of the event. For instance, clinic care is often characterized as being fragmented, and lacking in coordination and consistency of health care providers (Peznecker, 1984). These elements of unpredictability may influence women's decision making regarding the sterilization and feelings about the operative experience. It is reported in the NSFG studies of 1982 and 1988 that poor women, African American women, those not covered by insurance, and those who have not completed high school are far more likely to use publicly funded clinics to obtain their family planning services (Mosher & Pratt, 1990). Nine percent of women aged 15 to 44 depend on Medicaid for maternity health care expenses and another 17% have no insurance, private or public (Gold & Kenney, 1985). In addition 39% of physicians nationally who perform tubal sterilizations (49% in metropolitan areas) do not accept Medicaid or reduce their fees for low-income women (Orr et al., 1985). At costs ranging from $1,100 to $2,200 (reported in

1990 dollars), publicly funded clinics will be the only option for many women (Torres & Forrest, 1983).

Additionally, it is possible that women may be unprepared for the amount of postoperative pain they may feel. In recent years tubal sterilization has been called "Band-aid surgery" because the umbilical laparoscopic incision requires only a few sutures and a Band-aid. Many sterilizations are performed on an outpatient basis wherein the woman is hospitalized only long enough to undergo the procedure and recover from anesthesia, approximately 3 hours total (Greenspan et al., 1984). Increased nausea and vomiting during the 24 hours after surgery has been found to occur if the sterilization procedure occurred within the first 8 days of the menstrual cycle (Beattie et al., 1993). Post-sterilization pain may be due to carbon dioxide used to inflate the abdomen during the procedure that remains trapped under the diaphragm for up to 3 days (Hodgson, McClelland, & Newton, 1970). Pain often increases the first postoperative day, decreasing only slowly over subsequent days (Dobbs et al., 1987). Lower abdominal pain also occurs and is possibly due to ischemia of the fallopian tubes (Chi & Cole, 1979). One study found that if lidocaine were injected into the peritoneal space and the mesosaphinx of the tubes, postoperative pain was significantly less (Benhamou et al., 1994). If endometrial ablation has been performed along with the sterilization procedure, there might be an additional risk of long-term pain (Townsend et al., 1993). Six women with complaints of long-term pain were found to have endometrial scarring, and swollen fallopian tubes, to as much as twice their normal size. Thus, undergoing sterilization may be physically painful and the pain may continue after hospital discharge.

In addition, about 43% of sterilizations are performed during the postpartum period when the fallopian tubes are still adjacent to the umbilicus and readily accessible (Torres & Forrest, 1983). Since this period is also a time when women may feel emotionally labile (O'Hara, 1987), postoperative pain and/or emotional sequelae may be particularly difficult.

WOMEN'S RESPONSES TO TUBAL STERILIZATION

Many studies have been made of women's post-sterilization responses. Some have been considered in terms of psychiatric illness, but most have concerned requests for reversal and statements of regret. No relationship has been found between onset of psychiatric illness or suicide and sterilization (Vessey et al., 1983; WHO Collaborative Prospective

Study, 1984; 1985). A desire for reversal may indicate unhappiness with having undergone sterilization, but it may also mean a change in circumstances, such as remarriage and the desire for more children. Several studies have shown that women who were younger at the time of their first and last births and at the time of sterilization were more likely to be seeking reversal (Divers, 1984; Gomel, 1978; Leader et al., 1983; Thranov, Hertz, & Ryttov, 1987).

Studies of satisfaction with sterilization and regret have been problematic. In studies of the desire for reversal, investigators may select a control group of women previously sterilized who have not requested reversal. These women are then assumed to be satisfied, but this may not be the case. Maracil-Gratton (1988) found that 21% had felt regret at some stage after the procedure, but had not informed a physician. Another study found that of women requesting reversal, over 50% regretted their sterilization within 1 year, 26% within 2 years, and 21% after 2 years (Leader et al., 1983). There is little data on ethnicity and socioeconomic status (SES) and feelings about sterilization, but fewer years of education and lower SES have been reported.

Factors associated with making the sterilization decision may also be related to women's feelings. Being sterilized at the same time as a cesarean birth was found to increase the risk of regret compared to those being sterilized at a time unrelated to childbearing (Grubb et al., 1985). This may be a condition of forced choice, where the decision is made before the outcome of the pregnancy is known, and where the procedure is being performed to avoid subsequent surgery. Similarly, some studies have found a weak relationship between sterilizations performed during the postpartum period and feelings of regret or a desire for reversal afterwards (Divers, 1984; Grubb et al., 1985).

It was also found in a national study of sterilization effects conducted by the Center for Disease Control, that sterilized women had a history of using a higher number of contraceptive methods than did nonsterilized women. A higher percentage of sterilized women also had used barrier, rhythm, or withdrawal methods suggesting that they had exhausted the more reliable methods of contraception. Similarly, it was found in a study of childless women, who intended to remain childless, that they did not plan sterilization if they were satisfied with their contraceptive method (Callon & Hee, 1984).

The term regret has been poorly defined. It may indicate sad feelings about having undergone sterilization, the desire or wish for a(nother) baby, or the actual intention to have a(nother) baby if it were possible. Women might mean that they would not be sterilized again if they could do it over, that they regretted they could no longer have children but still believed it was the right decision, or that they wanted to have the procedure undone.

There is a body of literature concerning studies of menstrual changes after sterilization, but findings are mixed (Lethbridge, 1992).* It is possible that sterilization procedures jeopardize ovarian vascularity or promote endometriosis. Histologic findings of previously sterilized fallopian tubes have shown significantly more epithelial inclusions in fallopian tubes sterilized with rings, ligation, and coagulation, and focal endometriosis after tubal ligation and coagulation (Donnez et al., 1984). Additionally, disruption of the utero-ovarian blood supply may result in ovarian dysfunction, since the ovarian artery and vein run posterior to and closely parallel to the fallopian tube. Procedures that cause more tissue destruction such as tubal ligation or electrocoagulation might be more likely to affect vascularity than application of rings or clips.

In a study of 10,040 women for up to 2 years post-sterilization, the majority reported no change in their menses (Bhiwandiwala, Mumford, & Feldblum, 1983). Approximately 30% reported a change in some aspect of their menstrual cycles, but these were not necessarily negative. Previous contraceptive use was taken into account, since those who had used hormonal contraception prior to the sterilization reported a decrease in menstrual regularity and an increase in cycle length, flow duration and amount, and dysmenorrhea. Similarly, for those who discontinued use of the IUD, more women became regular and experienced a decrease in flow duration, amount of flow, dysmenorrhea, and midcycle bleeding. A study that correlated luteal phase hormonal levels and perimenstrual syndrome (PMS), however, found no differences in women who had undergone sterilization and a matched group that had not (Rojansky & Halbreich, 1991). There has not been definitive evidence, however that gonadal-ovarian hormones are responsible for PMS.

There is some evidence that menstrual disturbances might be more likely as time passes. In a long-term study with a control group, the group having been sterilized had significantly increased (i.e., nearly three times more) prevalence of abnormal cycles between 49 and 87 months after the procedure (DeStefano et al., 1985). Another long-term study of 5,070 women conducted by the Collaborative Review of Sterilization, found that 5 years after sterilization, 35% of the participants reported a high level of pain during menstruation, 49% had a heavy or very heavy menstrual flow, and 10% had spotting between menstrual

---

*From Lethbridge, D. J. (1992). Post tubal sterilization syndrome. *IMAGE: Journal of Nursing Scholarship, 24,* 15–18. Copyrighted material used by permission of Sigma Theta Tau International.

periods (Wilcox et al., 1992). In contrast, one year after sterilization, only 27% reported high levels of menstrual pain, 41% had a heavier flow, and 7% had spotting. Differences in methods were also significantly related. Those having had coagulation reported the longest and most irregular cycles, while those who had the spring clip had the shortest. The spring clip was also associated with increased bleeding the first three days of menstruation. This study was controlled for age, previous birth control use, and presterilization menstrual history. Other studies have found an increased risk of hysterectomy after tubal sterilization, when women were matched with controls (Goldhaber et al., 1993; Shy et al., 1992). This risk increased over time, and was not found to be related to the type of sterilization procedure used, suggesting that a biologic reason for the increased numbers of hysterectomies could not be supported by the data.

STERILIZATION REVERSAL

Sterilization reversal is usually performed by laparotomy and microsurgical techniques, and treatment with antibiotics and steroids. Success rates, meaning a pregnancy successfully carried to term, have been reported to range from 45 to 79% (Sauer et al., 1987). Characteristics considered necessary for a successful result include that there be no physical nor psychosocial contraindications to pregnancy, at least 4 cm of fallopian tube remain on at least one side, with intact fimbriae, biphasic basal body temperature charts are demonstrated with luteal-phase progesterone levels of over 5 ng/ml, and a hysterosalpingogram shows a normal uterine cavity. Partner characteristics include at least 20 million sperm/ml with 50% normally formed, 60% motility, and a postcoital test demonstrating at least five motile and progressive sperm per high-power field.

From 2 to 8% of women who have been sterilized seek reversal, and of that group only some 50% of reversals result in a term birth (Sauer et al., 1987). Sterilization is very costly and generally not covered by health insurance. One study reported that if a minilaparotomy was used, costs could be reduced to approximately $5,000 for the procedure (Daniell & McTavish, 1995).

VASECTOMY

Over half a million vasectomies are performed in the United States each year (Marquette et al., 1995). It is considered a very effective method of contraception, having a failure rate of approximately 1%. It is considerably less expensive than tubal sterilization, with costs ranging from $250 to $1,000.

PROCEDURE

Vasectomies are generally done under local anesthesia, through a one centimeter incision, or two incisions, one to locate each vas. The seminal cord is incised, and the vas deferens is clasped. A one centimeter portion may be excised and the ends then ligated and/or cauterized. The incision(s) are then closed through absorbable sutures. Thirty percent of men have been shown to experience vagal effects, such as diaphoresis, pallor, tachycardia, or fainting, through manipulation of the vas. It is not unusual for preoperative sedation to be given. One group of physicians suggests that a prepubic approach was useful, in that it gave easier access to the vas, healing was more rapid, and complications to the scrotum did not occur (Khanna et al., 1991).

COMPLICATIONS OF VASECTOMY

The most common complications of vasectomy are short-term, such as postoperative pain, hematoma, and infection (Alderman, 1991). Pain after the procedure will vary according to the man's tolerance, but it is frequently discussed in the literature and medical textbooks as discomfort or slight, which may be controlled with acetaminophen. One study suggested, however, that 77% of men reported pain and swelling after the first 24 hours, and 32% had complaints for 3 weeks (Rose, Kay, & Windfeld, 1991). Pain often occurs at the first attempt of sexual intercourse, possibly due to epididymal pressure or peristalsis in the proximal vas deferens, which is distended. However, long-term testicular pain has also been reported (McMahon et al., 1992). In this study, 33% reported long-term pain, but only 15% considered it troublesome and only three men reported they regretted the vasectomy because of long-term pain.

Hematomas will occur unless hemostasis has been very well controlled during the procedure. Any blood seepage during the procedure, or after, will not be well absorbed because of the loose tissue of the scrotum. Leg elevation, good scrotal support, and cold compresses help to reduce bleeding. However, the man must be warned that if the scrotum rapidly increases in size, he may need to have a hematoma evacuated and bleeding controlled. A hematoma will increase both pain and recovery time.

Wound infections are not uncommon, and will present with reddening and possible oozing. A deep infection or abscess will need to be cultured and treated with heat and antibiotics. Postoperative orchitis and epididymitis may also occur and are secondary to extravasation of sperm. The proximal vas and the epididymis will swell with backed-up sperm and it is difficult to distinguish between congestive epididymitis and true infection. Treatments include both anti-inflammatory drugs and antibiotics.

Possibly the most serious long-term complication is spontaneous recanalization. These are most common within 3 months after surgery and can occur up to a year after. Factors increasing the incidence of recanalization include: sperm granulomas, removal of less than one centimeter of vas, insufficient cauterization of one or both ends of the vas, and the development of a deep abscess. It is imperative that men undergo semen analysis after the procedure. In one study, however, only 26% of men returned the two or more samples suggested following surgery (Smucker et al., 1991). In this group, 45% had not returned any samples and reported that the inconvenience and embarrassment hampered their compliance. The men who had not returned any samples were more likely to report that their partners would not be very upset if the vasectomy failed and pregnancy resulted, but since only the men were interviewed, this suggestion must be considered as only tentative.

A sperm granuloma is a small nodule that may be palpable at the proximal end of the resected vas. They are generally 3 to 5 mm in size, but may be considerably larger. The incidence of sperm granulomas forming is 20 to 25% of men. It is an inflammatory reaction to extravasated sperm. The granuloma contains masses of sperm surrounded by epithelial cells and connective tissue. Epithelial-lined channels form that may contain sperm and spermiophages, and lymphocytes. Small canaliculi form, and may be adequate to connect the two ends of the resected vas. Sperm granulomas should be suspected if a man complains of pain and swelling at the vasectomy site 1 or 2 weeks after surgery, especially if there has been a pain-free period. A vasitis nodosa may also occur and is a predecessor to recanalization. It may form shortly after the procedure, but unlike sperm granulomas, may also occur years later. A vasitis nodosa forms as blind channels lined with epithelium of the vasal lumen on the proximal end. As the vasitis nodosa progresses, the channels may result in ductules, eventually joining with the distal end of the vas.

Immunological changes have been found to occur as the body absorbs unejaculated sperm. Since mature sperm are not present until puberty, absorbed sperm are treated as foreign bodies and antibodies form. Sixty to eighty percent of men have been found to have serum sperm antibodies following vasectomy (Hellema & Rümke, 1978). While there has been evidence of increased atherosclerosis in monkeys, no evidence has been found in humans for increased cardio-vascular problems related to circulating antibodies (Massey et al., 1984; Walker et al., 1983). There have been mixed findings related to the increased possibility of prostatic cancer after vasectomy. Studies showing a higher incidence have had methodological deficiencies, and other studies have shown no effect.

REVERSAL OF VASECTOMY

Studies of men requesting vasectomy reversal suggest that it is more likely in cases of a change in marital status, where newly single men feel disadvantaged because of their infertility or a new partner desires a pregnancy. It is also more likely in those who were younger at the time of vasectomy, and had the procedure during a time of emotional crisis (Clarke & Gregson, 1986). Success rates, meaning a successful pregnancy carried to term, have not been more than approximately 50% (Hendry, 1994). Difficulties have been related to microsurgical technique, where sperm leakage has occurred through a suture line and granuloma formation has led to secondary obstruction. The sperm count rises slowly after reversal and usually reaches a plateau by 6 months. Time since the vasectomy seems to be a factor in success rates, in that success rates of 76%, if fewer than 3 years, 53% after 3 to 8 years, 44% after 9 to 14 years, and 30% after more than 15 years (Belker et al., 1989). Other factors predicting success include spermatozoa found in the proximal vas. An absence suggests secondary changes may have taken place in the epididymis. Vasectomy increases pressure in the proximal end of the vas which is transferred to the epididymis. Rupture of tubules in the epididymis may occur, causing obstruction. Vasectomy may also cause damage to adjacent nerves near the vas and the epididymis, affecting ejaculator ability. Finally, there is suggestion that the number or nature of antisperm antibodies may affect success. One study found serum antibodies in 48% of men whose partners had successful pregnancies, and 94% of those men whose partners did not (Sullivan & Howe, 1977). Very high serum titres may relate to continued infertility. If the antibodies are classed as IgA, like those found in spontaneously infertile men (Parslow et al., 1983), they are more likely to cause infertility post-vasectomy. A study of antibody characteristics showed those men with pure IgG response had an 86% pregnancy success rate; those with IgG and IgA together had a 43% success rate; those with IgA only had a 22% success rate, and it fell to 0 when there was only IgA and a strong immune response as well (Meinertz et al., 1990).

STRATEGIES FOR INTERVENTION

Providers and other health care personnel are involved with women and men undergoing sterilization, during decision making, throughout the procedures in operating rooms, and for aftercare on surgical floors, outpatient clinics or postpartum units. Many women and men with a history of sterilization are clients for subsequent health care. Comprehensive care would include ensuring that individuals and couples making the decision to undergo sterilization are fully informed of the procedure and possible sequelae and, in light of its stated permanence, have considered the alternatives to sterilization. Ideally, follow-up care would include checking for compliance for postoperative instructions, such as the return of semen samples after vasectomy to ensure that the surgery was successful. Finally, adjustment to sterilization must be monitored with recovery over time.

Specific postoperative care after tubal sterilization includes:

1. Women are often unprepared for the pain they will feel postoperatively since the surgical procedure is so often minimized. They should have effective oral analgesia to take home, with instructions for taking it, especially if they are breastfeeding. They should call their health care provider if the pain is severe.
2. No lifting or vigorous exercise for 1–2 weeks.
3. Showering rather than bathing for a week.
4. If done postpartum, help will be needed at home with other children.
5. Sterilization is immediate and sexual activity without other contraception may resume as soon as comfortable.

Postoperative care after vasectomy includes:

1. Keep feet elevated and apply ice to the groin to reduce swelling and bleeding. Bruising will be present for approximately two weeks.
2. Use an athletic supporter until he is comfortable without it.
3. Take pain medication as needed. Call his health care provider if pain becomes severe.

4. Do not engage in lifting or vigorous exercise for two to three days or until comfortable.
5. Shower rather than bathing.
6. Possible reactions include infection—redness, swelling, tenderness, fever, or oozing of pus; more than a small amount of swelling; a granuloma forming over the incision. If it is larger than ½ inch, see his health care provider.
7. Sexual activity may resume when comfortable, and may begin one or two times the first week, increasing to as desired after three weeks. The use of contraception is necessary during sexual intercourse, since sperm will still be present in the distal vas.
8. Two semen checks are necessary to confirm sterilization. The first should be done 6 weeks after surgery or after 15 ejaculations; the second after 3 months. Contraception must be used until the ejaculate is free of sperm.

Teaching in preparation for tubal sterilization and vasectomy should include:

1. A thorough history should be obtained, including age of the man and his partner, marital status and number of children, occupation and education of the woman or man and the partner, history of previous marriages, condition and length of the current marital relationship and sexual functioning, and the purpose of seeking sterilization.

2. The couples' decision-making process should be explored. How long have they considered having the procedure? Are they under any particular stress? Are there moral or religious conflicts? Has he had friends or acquaintances undergo the procedure and what were their experiences? Have they considered all alternatives?

3. During a health assessment for the man, a history of previous intrascrotal surgery, infections, or trauma or other possible causes of altered anatomy or formation of adhesions should be noted. Health assessment for the woman should include a history of reproductive physiological anomalies, abdominal adhesion formation, pelvic inflammatory disease or pelvic trauma. Major illnesses such as a bleeding disorder, diabetes, coronary artery disease, epilepsy or psychiatric disorder should also be assessed, as well as medication use such as anticoagulants, aspirin, insulin, beta blockers, nitroglycerin, anticonvulsants, or tranquilizers.

4. Thorough teaching and preparation would include teaching the man and his partner male reproductive anatomy and physiology such that they understand what will occur during the vasectomy; where the

sperm is manufactured and what will now happen to it; the role of testosterone and the lack of effect of vasectomy on it, as well as a distinction between "castration" and vasectomy; and the continuation of normal sexual functioning and minimally changed ejaculate. For the woman, reproductive anatomy and physiology of external and internal organs, including that ovarian function and hormonal levels will continue, that ova will be released but reabsorbed, and that menses generally continue unchanged. A man undergoing vasectomy or a woman undergoing tubal sterilization should be prepared for the possibility of any complications and actions to take.

REFERENCES

Alderman, P. (1991). Complications in a series of 1224 vasectomies. *The Journal of Family Practice, 33,* 579–584.

Bachrach, C., Horn, M., Mosher, W., & Shimizu, I.(1985). National survey of family growth, Cycle III, sample design, weighing and variance estimation. *Vital and Health Statistics,* Series 2, No. 98.

Balakrishnan, T. R., Krotki, K., & Lapaierre-Adamcyk, E. (1985). Contraceptive use in Canada, 1984. *Family Planning Perspectives, 17,* 209–215.

Beattie, W. S., Lindblad, T., Buckley, D. N., & Forrest, J. B. (1993). Menstruation increases the risk of nausea and vomiting after laparoscopy: A prospective randomized study. *Anesthesiology, 78*(2), 272–276.

Benhamou, D., Narchi, P., Mazoit J. X., & Fernandez, H. (1994). Postoperative pain after local anesthetics for laparoscopic sterilization. *Obstetrics and Gynecology, 84*(5), 877–880.

Bhiwandiwala, P. P., Mumford, S. D., & Feldblum, P. J. (1983). Menstrual pattern changes following laparoscopic sterilization with different occlusion techniques: A review of 10,004 cases. *American Journal of Obstetrics and Gynecology, 145,* 684–694.

Callon, V. J., & Hee, R. W. Q. (1984). The choice of sterilization: voluntarily childless couples, mothers of one child by choice, and males seeking reversal of vasectomy. *Journal of Biosocial Science, 16,* 241–248.

Chen, T. F., & Ball, R. Y. (1991). Epididymectomy for post-vasectomy pain: Histological review. *British Journal of Urology, 68*(4), 407–413.

Chi, I.-C., & Cole, L. P. (1979). Incidence of pain among women undergoing laparoscopic sterilization by electrocoagulation, the spring loaded clip, and tubal ring. *American Journal of Obstetrics and Gynecology, 135,* 397–401.

Clarke, L., & Gregson, S. (1986). Who has a vasectomy reversal? *Journal of Biosocial Science, 18,* 253–259.

Daniell, J. F., & McTavaish, G. (1995). Combined laparoscopy and mini-laparotomy for outpatient reversal of tubal sterilization. *Southern Medical Journal, 88*(9), 914–916.

DeStefano, F., Perlman, J. A., Peterson, H. B., & Diamond, E. L. (1985). Long-term risk of menstrual disturbances after tubal sterilization. *American Journal of Obstetrics and Gynecology, 152,* 835–841.

DeVilliers, V. P., & Morkel, D. J. (1987). Postpartum sterilization by the Irving technique. *South African Medical Journal, 71,* 253.

Divers, W. A. (1984). Characteristics of women requesting reversal of sterilization. *Fertility and Sterility, 41,* 233–236.

Dobbs, F. F., Kumar, V., Alexander, J. I., & Hull, M. G. R. (1987). Pain after laparoscopy related to posture and ring versus clip steriliza-tion. *British Journal of Obstetrics and Gynecology, 94,* 262–266.

Donnez, J., Casanas-Roux, F., Ferin, J., & Thomas, K. (1984). Tubal polyps, epithelial inclusions and endometriosis after tubal steril-ization. *Fertility and Sterility, 41,* 564–568.

Dwyer, J. C., & Haws, J. M. (1990). Is permanent contraception accept-able in subSaharan Africa? *Studies in Family Planning, 21,* 322–326.

Gold, R. B., & Kenney, A. M. (1985). Paying for maternity care. *Family Planning Perspectives, 17,* 103–111.

Goldhabaer, M. K., Armstrong, M. A., Golditch, I. M., Sheehe, P. R., Petitti, D. B., & Friedman, G. D. (1993). Long-term risk of hysterec-tomy among 80,007 sterilized and comparison women at Kaiser Permanente, 1971–1987. *American Journal of Epidemiology, 138*(7), 508–521.

Gomel, V. (1978). Profile of women requesting reversal of sterilization. *Fertility and Sterility, 30,* 39–41.

Greenspan, J. R., Phillips, J. M., Rubin, G. L., Rhodenhiser, E. P., & Ory, H. W. (1984). Tubal sterilizations performed in freestanding, ambu-latory-care surgical facilities in the United States in 1980. *Journal of Reproductive Medicine, 29,* 237–241.

Griffin, W. T., & Mandsager, N. T. (1987). Spring clip sterilization: Long-term follow-up. *Southern Medical Journal, 80,* 301–304.

Grubb, G. S., Peterson, H. B., Layde, P. M., & Rubin, G. L. (1985). Regret after the decision to have a tubal sterilization. *Fertility and Sterility, 44,* 248–253.

Hellema, H. W., & Rümke, P. (1978). Immune sperm agglutination: are only motile spermatozoa involved? *Clinical and Experimental Immu-nology, 31*(1) 12–17.

Hendry, W. F. (1994). Vasectomy and vasectomy reversal. *British Journal of Urology, 73,* 337–344.

Hirschowitz, L., Rode, J., Guillebaud, J., Bounds, W., & Moss, E. (1988).

Vasitis nodosa and associated clinical findings. *Journal of Clinical Pathology, 41,* 419–423.

Hodgson, C., McClelland, R. M. A., & Newton, J. R. (1970). Some effects of the peritoneal insufflation of carbon dioxide at laparoscopy. *Anaesthesia, 25,* 382–390.

Irving, F. C. (1950). Tubal sterilization. *American Journal of Obstetrics and Gynecology, 60,* 1101–1106.

Khanna, Y. K., Khanna, A., Heda, K. R., Mathur, G., & Jhanji, R. N. (1991). Pre-pubic vasectomy—a new approach. *Postgraduate Medicine, 37*(2), 65–68.

Leader, A., Galan, N., George, R., & Taylor, P. J. (1983). A comparison of definable traits in women requesting reversal of sterilization and women satisfied with sterilization. *American Journal of Obstetrics and Gynecology, 145,* 198–202.

Lethbridge, D. J. (1992). Post-tubal sterilization syndrome. *Image: Journal of Nursing Scholarship, 24,* 15–18.

Marcil-Gratton, N. (1988). Sterilization regret among women in metropolitan Montreal. *Family Planning Perspectives, 20,* 222–227.

Marquette, C. M., Koonin, L. M., Antarsh, L., Gargiullo, P. M., & Smith, J. C. (1995). Vasectomy in the United States, 1991. *American Journal of Public Health, 85*(5), 644–649.

Massey, F. J., Bernstein, G. S., O'Fallon, W. M., Schuman, L. M., Cowlson, A. H., Crozier, R., Mandel, J. S., Benjamin, R. B., Berendes, H. W., Chang, P. C., Detels, R., Ernslander, R. F., Korelitz, J., Kurland, L. T., Lepow, I. H., McGregor, D. D., Nakamura, R. N., Quiroga, J., Schmidt, S., Spivey, G. H., & Sullivan, T. (1984). Vasectomy and health: Results from a large cohort study. *Journal of the American Medical Association, 252,* 1023–1030.

McMahon, A. J., Buckley, J., Taylor, A., Lloyd, S. N., Deane, R. F. & Kirk, D. (1992). Chronic testicular pain following vasectomy. *British Journal of Urology, 69*(2), 188–191.

Meinertz, H., Linnet, L., Andersen, P. F., & Hjort, T. (1990). Antisperm antibodies and fertility after vasovasostomy: a follow-up study of 216 men. *Fertility and Sterility, 54,* 315–321.

Mexico National Survey on Fertility and Health (1990). Mexico 1987: Results from the demographic and health survey. *Studies in Family Planning, 21,* 181–185.

Mosher, W. D., & Pratt, W. F. (1990). Contraceptive use in the United States, 1973–1988. *Advance data from vital and health statistics, No. 182.* Hyattsville, MD: National Center for Health Statistics.

O'Hara, M. W. (1987). Post-partum "blues," depression, and psychosis: A review. *Journal of Psychosomatic Obstetrics and Gynecology, 7,* 205–227.

Orr, M. R., Forrest, J. D., Johnson, J. H., & Tolman, D. L. (1985). The provision of sterilization services by private physicians. *Family Planning Perspectives, 17,* 216–220.

Parslow, J. M., Royle, M. G., Kingscorr, M. M. B., Wallace, D. M. A., & Hendry, W. F. (1983). The effects of sperm antibodies on fertility after vasectomy reversal. *American Journal of Reproductive Immunology, 3,* 28–31.

Peterson, H. B., Hulka, J. F., Spielman, F. J., Lee, S., & Marachbanks, P. A. (1987). Local versus general anesthesia for laparoscopic sterilization: A randomized study. *Obstetrics and Gynecology, 70,* 903–908.

Peznecker, B. L. (1984). The poor: A population at risk. *Public Health Nursing, 1,* 237–249.

Poston, Jr., D. L. (1986). Patterns of contraceptive use in China. *Studies in Family Planning, 17,* 217–227.

Rojansky, N., & Halbreich, U. (1991). Prevalence and severity of premenstrual changes after tubal sterilization. *Journal of Reproductive Medicine, 36*(8), 551–555.

Rose, M., Kay, L., & Windfeld, M. (1991). Rekonvalescens efter ambulant vasektomi [Recovery after ambulatory vasectomy]. *Ugeskr Laeger (Denmark), 153*(27), 1943–1945.

Sauer, M. V., Zeffin, K. B., Bustillo, M. C., & Buster, J. E. (1987). Sterilization reversals performed by fellows in training: What success rates can we reasonably expect? *Microsurgery, 8,* 125–127.

Shy, K. K., Stergachis, A., Grothaus, L. G., Wagner, E. H., Hecht, J., & Anderson, F. (1992). Tubal sterilization and risk of subsequent hospital admission for menstrual disorders. *American Journal of Obstetrics and Gynecology, 166*(6, Pt. 1), 16989–1705.

Sullivan, M. J., & Howe, G. E. (1977). Correlation for circulating antisperm antibodies to functional success in vasovasostomy. *Journal of Urology, 117,* 189–191.

Thailand Demographic and Health Survey. (1989). Thailand 1987: Results from the Demographic and Health Survey. *Studies in Family Planning, 20,* 62–66.

Thranov, I., Hertz, J., & Ryttov, N. (1987). Profile of Danish women undergoing reversal of sterilization, 1978–1983. *Acta Obset Gynecol Scand, 66,* 269–273.

Townsend, D. E., McCausland, V., McCausland, A., Fields, G., & Kauffman, K. (1993). Post-ablation tubal sterilization syndrome. *Obstetrics and Gynecology, 82*(3), 422–424.

Walker, A. M., Jick, H., Hunter, J. R., & McEvoy, J. (1983). Vasectomy and non-fatal myocardial infarction: continued observations indicates no elevation of risk. *Journal of Urology, 130,* 936–937.

Wilcox, L. S., Martinez-Schnell, B., Peterson, H. B., Ware, J. H., & Hughes, J. M. (1992). Menstrual function after tubal sterilization. *American Journal of Epidemiology, 135*(12), 1368–1381.

World Health Organization Collaborative Prospective Study. (1984). Mental health and female sterilization. *Journal of Biosocial Science, 17,* 1–21.

World Health Organization Collaborative Prospective Study. (1985). Mental health and female sterilization: A follow-up. *Journal of Biosocial Science, 18,* 1–18.

World Health Organization Task Force on Female Sterilization. (1982). Mini-incision for postpartum sterilization of women: A multi-centered multinational prospective study. *Contraception, 26,* 495–503.

Yoon, I. B., & Poliakoff, S. F. (1978). Laparoscopic tubal ligation: A follow-up report on the Yoon Falope-Ring methodology. *Journal of Reproductive Medicine, 23,* 76–80.

Index

Index

barriers to use of, 162
beliefs and perceptions of, 161–163
benefits of, 157–159, 162
breakage and slippage of, 163–164
choice of, 158–159
cost of, 11–12
for disease prevention, 29, 71, 91, 158
distribution in schools, 7
effectiveness of, 157
failure rate of, 116
female, 149
    and disease prevention, 158
instructions for use of, 159–161
natural membrane, 158–159, 164
perceptions of
    by female adolescents, 89
    by males, 73
polyurethane, 157, 159, 164
side effects of, 18
use by adolescents, 67–68, 82, 85
use by adults, 68–69
use by midlife women, 102
use rates for, 154–156
Copper-bearing IUDs, 199–201, 205–206
Costs
of contraceptives, 11–12
of tubal sterilization, 216
of vasectomy, 216
Creams, spermicidal, 144–145
Creighton program for teaching natural family planning, 173, 180
Cultural beliefs
American, compared to other countries, 53–54
and contraceptive choice and use, 4–6, 32, 52–58
on sexuality, 9
and socially undesirable pregnancies, 113

Dalkon Shield, 197–198
Decision making, contraceptive, 35–42
by female adolescents, 88–91

and hormonal contraceptive use, 124–129
male and female role in, 55
by males, 72
Depo-Provera use, warning signs for, 127–128
Diaphragms, 144–147
advantages and disadvantages of, 145
cost of, 12
disliked by Asian women, 52
failure rate of, 116
fitting of, 146–147
instructions for use of, 145–147
reported use of, 141
side effects of, 18
use in adolescence, 82
use by midlife women, 102
Disease prevention, *see* Sexually transmitted diseases
Douching as contraceptive method, 18, 26, 190–192
experimentation with, in adolescence, 85

Ectopic pregnancy
and hormonal contraceptive use, 123
and IUD use, 201–202
Education
about condom use, 159–161
about contraceptive methods, 9–10
about sexuality, in schools, 7
and female contraceptive use, 58, 68, 88
for hormonal contraceptive use, 124–128
information communication in, 38
information sources in, 71–72
for males, 71–72
for midlife women, 98
Efficacy of contraceptives
estimated by family planning practitioners, 114
life table calculations, 117
Pearl index of, 116–117

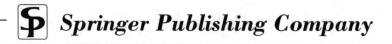

Ⓢ *Springer Publishing Company*

Psychological Aspects of Women's Reproductive Health

Michael W. O'Hara, PhD, Robert C. Reiter, MD, Susan R. Johnson, MD, Alison Milburn, PhD, and Jane Engeldinger, MD, Editors

In this insightful text, the editors explore the interrelationship between the psychology of women and their reproductive health. This volume will be of interest to psychiatrists, psychologists, and counselors, as well as nurses, social workers, and other health professionals and students concerned with mental health.

PSYCHOLOGICAL
ASPECTS *of*
WOMEN'S
REPRODUCTIVE
HEALTH

Michael W. O'Hara, PhD
Robert C. Reiter, MD
Susan R. Johnson, MD
Alison Milburn, PhD
Jane Engeldinger, MD
Editors

Ⓢ *Springer Publishing Company*

Contents:

I. Reproductive Transitions. Menstruation, *S.R. Johnson* • Childbearing, *M.W. O'Hara* • Menopause, *M.K. Walling*

II. Gynecology. Chronic Pelvic Pain, *M.K. Walling and R.C. Reiter* • Gynecologic Surgery, *A.F. Stockman* • Gynecologic Cancer, *L.A. Menefee* • Contraception, *K.K. Brewer* • Sexually Transmitted Diseases, *A. Milburn and K.K. Brewer*

III. Obstetrics. Infertility, *R.L. Davisson* • Prenatal Diagnosis, *G.L. Rose* • Childbirth Preparation, *E.F. Swanson-Hyland* • Pregnancy Loss Through Miscarriage or Stillbirth, *K.L. Cole* • Abortion, *E.A. Weerts Whitmore* • High-Risk Pregnancy, *L.L. Gorman* • Adolescent Pregnancy, *R.M. MacFarlane*

IV. Decision Making. Medical Decision Making, *C.J. Hodne*

1995   368pp   0-8261-8660-2   hardcover

536 Broadway, New York, NY 10012-3955 • (212) 431-4370 • Fax (212) 941-7842

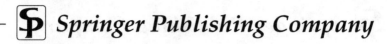
Springer Publishing Company

Psychosocial Adaptation in Pregnancy
Assessment of Seven Dimensions of Maternal Development, Second Edition
Regina P. Lederman, PhD, FAAN

A groundbreaking analysis of the psychology of pregnancy, now in a second edition. The author identifies seven distinct areas in which the most change and development occur during pregnancy, based on her in-depth interviews with pregnant women.

Original research on first-time mothers is presented along with information from the author's new research with mothers having subsequent children. The scholarly development of theory is intertwined with the "voices" of women describing the emotions experienced in pregnancy in their own words, making this a valuable resource for students, researchers, and clinicians in maternal-child health.

> **Psychosocial Adaptation in Pregnancy**
> Second Edition
> Assessment of Seven Dimensions of Maternal Development
>
> Regina P. Lederman

Contents:
- Acceptance of Pregnancy
- Identification with a Motherhood Role
- Relationship to Mother
- Relationship to Husband
- Preparation for Labor
- Prenatal Fear of Loss of Control in Labor
- Prenatal Fear of Self-Esteem in Labor
- Methods of Assessment
- Prenatal Adaptation Among Multigravidas

1996   336pp   0-8261-6710-1   hardcover

536 Broadway, New York, NY 10012-3955 • (212) 431-4370 • Fax (212) 941-7842

SP *Springer Publishing Company*

Becoming A Mother
Research on Maternal Role Identity From Rubin to the Present
Ramona T. Mercer, RN, PhD, FAAN

A comprehensive review of all the current knowledge on maternal role attainment since Reva Rubin's seminal work. Drawing from research in nursing, maternal-child health, psychology, sociology, and social work, this book examines the psychological transition to motherhood from a contemporary, multidisciplinary perspective. Special circumstances such as preterm birth and single parenthood are discussed, as well as the effect of maternal employment, and maternal age (such as teens and older mothers).

Contents:

I: Anticipating Motherhood. Feminine Identity and Maternal Behavior • Cognitive Work During Pregnancy • Maternal Tasks During Pregnancy

II: Achieving The Maternal Identity. Physical and Psychological Recovery Postpartum • The Process of Becoming Acquainted With/Attached to the Infant • Work Toward Maternal Competence Early Postpartum • Integrating the Maternal Self • Preterm Birth • Transition to the Maternal Role Following the Birth of an Infant with Anomalies or Chronic Illness

III: The Mother in Social Context. Life Circumstances and Teenage, Older, and Single Mothers • Employment and the Maternal Role

Springer Series: Focus on Women
1995 392pp 0-8261-8970-9 hardcover

536 Broadway, New York, NY 10012-3955 • (212) 431-4370 • Fax (212) 941-7842

Springer Publishing Company

Becoming A Father
Contemporary Social, Emotional, and Clinical Perspectives
Jerrold L. Shapiro, PhD, **Michael J. Diamond**, PhD, and **Martin Greenberg,** MD, Editors
Foreword: **T. Berry Brazelton**

One of the most important events in men's lives is becoming a father. This transition has life long psychological, social, and emotional effects. In this volume, the editors and contributors explore both the dramatic increase in the involvement of fathers in pregnancy, childbirth, and early parenting, as well as the implications of fatherhood from a sociocultural, psychodynamic, and personal perspective.

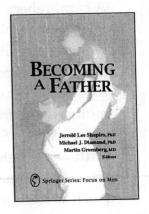

BECOMING A FATHER

Jerrold Lee Shapiro, PhD
Michael J. Diamond, PhD
Martin Greenberg, MD
Editors

Springer Series: Focus on Men

Partial Contents:

I. The Social Perspective. The Changing Role of Fathers, *M. Lamb* • The Paternal Presence, *K. Pruett* • Bringing in Fathers: The Reconstruction of Mothering, *D. Ehrensaft* • The Mother's Role in Promoting Fathering Behavior, *P. Jordan* • When Men Are Pregnant, *J. Shapiro* • Support for Fathers: A Model For Hospital-Based Parenting Programs, *P. Shecket* • Fatherhood, Numbness, and Emotional Self-Awareness, *R. Levant* • Teaching Responsible Fathering, *C. Ballard & M. Greenberg* • Teen Fathers: The Search for the Father, *M. Greenberg & H. Brown*

II. Personal Perspective. Three Tries To Get It Right, *L. Peltz* • Essay for Father's Day, *L. Kutner* • The New Father and The Old: Understanding the Relational Struggle of Fathers, *S. Osherson* • The Father Wound: Implications for Expectant Fathers, *J. Pleck* • Engrossment Revisited, *A. Bader*

III. The Clinical Perspective. Shifting Patterns of Fathering in the First Year of Life, *J. Hyman* • Becoming a Father, *M. Diamond* • Some Reflections on Adaptive Grandiosity in Fatherhood,*P. Wolson* • A Delicate Balance, *W. Pollack* • During the Transition to Fatherhood, *B. Sachs*

Springer Series: Focus on Men
1995   408pp   0-8261-8400-6   hardcover

536 Broadway, New York, NY 10012-3955 • (212) 431-4370 • Fax (212) 941-7842